NANNY OR STEWARD?

The role of government in public health

Karen Jochelson

In the past year, there has been much debate over the government's role in public health issues such as smoking and obesity. Is government intervention in these areas an example of 'nanny statism' – an unnecessary intrusion into people's lives? Or is it a form of 'stewardship' – part of government's responsibility to protect national health? This paper looks at the options open to governments that want to influence individual and collective behaviour to reduce health risks. It also examines historical and contemporary evidence on the impact of state intervention on public health.

Published by:

King's Fund
11–13 Cavendish Square
London W1G 0AN
www.kingsfund.org.uk

© King's Fund 2005

Charity registration number: 207401

First published 2005

ISBN 1 85717 538 7

A catalogue record for this publication is available from the British Library.

Available from:

King's Fund
11–13 Cavendish Square
London W1G 0AN
Tel: 020 7307 2591
Fax: 020 7307 2801
Email: publications@kingsfund.org.uk
www.kingsfund.org.uk/publications

Edited by: Lyn Whitfield and Lucy Latchmore
Typeset by: Peter Powell Origination & Print Limited
Printed in Great Britain by the King's Fund

Contents

List of figures

About the author

Karen Jochelson is a Fellow in Health Policy at the King's Fund. She is interested in the relationship between health and the physical and social environment. Her work on lifestyle change looks at the impact of government regulation on population health, personal decision-making and health, and consumer marketing in public health. Her work on sustainable development, public health and the NHS has looked at corporate citizenship, public sector procurement of hospital foods, better designed, healthier NHS buildings, and the management of energy, waste and transport. Karen previously worked as a consultant on sustainability and corporate responsibility projects in the private and public sectors in Europe and the United States. She has published extensively on health, HIV, racism, business and politics.

Acknowledgements

I would like to thank Clare Delap and Sally Norwood for help with the research, and Tony Harrison, Anna Coote, Jennifer Dixon and Virginia Berridge for asking provocative questions.

Karen Jochelson
October 2005

Introduction

The past year has seen some contentious debates about public health in the United Kingdom, focusing on a ban on smoking in public places, food labelling and food advertising to children. Some people have argued that any government intervention in these areas is 'nanny statist' – an unnecessary intrusion into people's lives and what they do, eat and drink. Others have argued that only the state can effectively reduce the poverty that is so often the root cause of ill health.

This is not a new debate; it has been held many times in the past, sometimes over government interventions that are now widely supported, or pass without comment. Dismissing government intervention as nanny statist is not particularly helpful when thinking about the options open to government and their likely impact. This paper suggests that there is a strong argument to be made for government intervention to safeguard public health. Legislation brings about changes that individuals on their own cannot, and sets new standards for the public good. Rather than condemning such activity as nanny statist, it might be more appropriate to view it as a form of 'stewardship'. Stewardship implies government has a responsibility for protecting national health, and to serve in the public interest and for the public good (Saltman and Ferroussier-Davis 2000). It suggests a protective function, where individuals are protected from harm by others and sometimes from themselves. Stewardship implies that paternalistic government is acceptable under certain conditions, and the debate should focus both on defining these conditions and the likely benefits.

The first part of this paper looks briefly at the options open to governments that want to influence individual and collective behaviour to reduce health risks. It then examines the 'nanny state' debate, looking at examples from the past and today. It looks at how government views its activities, and what opinion polls tell us about public views of government intervention.

The second part of this paper looks at historical and contemporary evidence on the impact of state intervention on public health through case studies on alcohol, smoking and road safety. The case studies suggest that higher taxes, advertising bans, and regulations backed with penalties encourage healthier behaviour by shaping the context in which people make decisions. Education and information programmes complement regulatory or fiscal interventions, and over time change individual attitudes and social norms. However, on their own they do not persuade people to behave differently.

The final part draws some conclusions about the role of government, the impact of government intervention, and the nature of stewardship.

The King's Fund has a longstanding commitment to improving the health of communities, particularly those that are disadvantaged. Our current public health programme, *Finding the Balance: Government, individuals and public health*, explores the relationship between government intervention and individual responsibility, trying to define the limits, benefits and drawbacks of both. We suggest that the nanny-state debate too quickly ignores the potential health benefits of government intervention. Understanding how government regulation creates a context in which individuals can make healthier choices is an important part of the debate.

Part 1: Government or individuals – whose responsibility is health?

Concern about new 'epidemics' of obesity, binge drinking and sexually transmitted disease has pushed public health up the policy agenda in the past few years. The second Wanless report (2004) suggested that the government needed to find cost-effective ways of preventing ill health and that public health intervention was crucial to developing a population 'fully engaged' in living healthy lives. The White Paper *Choosing Health: Making healthier choices easier* (Department of Health 2004) seeks to create demand for healthier lifestyles by providing more information and support for individuals, particularly those living in disadvantaged areas.

The media and the public have followed debates about how to persuade individuals to lead healthier lives with considerable interest. Health spokespeople for the three main political parties have clashed over the scope of a smoking ban in public places. Food is also a hot political topic, thanks to the school meals campaign launched by celebrity chef Jamie Oliver. Regional differences are also evident with Scotland introducing a total smoking ban and raising school food standards, and England lagging behind.

Any government that wants to change the behaviour of companies or the public in response to a perceived health risk has a number of policy options open to it. It can introduce measures that encourage change in individuals, such as public information campaigns or a new health promotion service. It can introduce enabling measures that promote change in populations, such as increasing or lowering taxation to encourage particular choices. Or it can introduce restrictive measures that ban or regulate activities or products, such as advertising codes, minimum food or air standards, or the compulsory wearing of seatbelts.

On some issues it seems self-evident that government intervention is most effective, as individuals on their own cannot effect significant social change. Air pollution is a good example. It took the London smog of December 1952, from which at least 4,000 people died, and the public furore and reports that followed, to persuade the government to finally pass the Clean Air Act of 1956. The Act controlled domestic and industrial sources of pollution for the first time (Brimblecombe 1987; Centre for History in Public Health 2002). Pollution levels were already declining before the smog, as consumers changed from coal to gas and electricity. But the Act had a significant impact. Domestic smoke emissions fell from about 1.35 million tonnes a year to 0.55 million tonnes and industrial smoke emissions from about 1 million to about 0.1 million tonnes between 1956 and 1971 (Ashby and Anderson 1981).

Reducing air pollution today means changing a country's travel infrastructure and spatial planning and energy policies. True, this requires that individuals make different choices, but this is most likely to happen when government makes it possible and influences people's choices. Creating a cheap and efficient public transport system, higher taxes on cars, petrol and road use, and spatial planning based on a public rather than private transport system, are most likely to change the way individuals travel and so affect air pollution and public health.

If government's role in controlling air pollution seems self-evident, then is its role any different when it comes to our eating, drinking, exercise and sexual habits? It seems so, as much of the recent public debate has focused on the idea of a 'nanny state', or whether it is legitimate for the government to intervene in people's personal lives. In the simplest terms, the protagonists of this debate can be described as interventionists and libertarians. For interventionists, governments promote freedom for individuals by creating opportunities and trying to even out inequities in society. For libertarians, minimal government is the best way to protect individual freedom, which is about not being interfered with by others.

Of course, there are many shades of grey between the two camps: libertarians will accept some forms of state intervention, recognising that this creates a framework for individual freedoms; and interventionists will draw the line at some state activities, believing they undermine individual rights and liberties. But the two positions help make sense of historical and contemporary debates about the limits to state action. The following section looks at historical and contemporary examples of the libertarian and interventionist debate. It looks at government views of its role, and what public opinion surveys tell us about popular views on individual and government responsibilities for health.

Historical antecedents

The debate over the limits to state intervention and extent of individual freedom has been played out many times in the past, and regulations we now take completely for granted sparked fierce controversy in their time:

The first British Public Health Act, passed in 1848, made local government responsible for the water and sewerage systems. Opposition to the Act came from defenders of local government autonomy who opposed the 'paternalist' and 'despotic interference' of national government into the lives of individuals and the free market. For one newspaper, 'a little dirt and freedom' was 'more desirable than no dirt at all and slavery' (Porter 1999).

The Licensing Act, 1872, restricted opening hours for pubs and prohibited children from drinking spirits in a pub. The drink trade regarded the Act as attacks on private property. Liberals felt they needed to protect the 'liberty of a few against the power of the many' and so felt it better that 'England should be free than... compulsorily sober'. Temperance supporters replied that 'drunken freedom' was 'not liberty' (Harrison 1971; Rose 1984).

The first attempts at legislation to control air pollution from domestic coal fires were stymied for 70 years. Critics believed that the public wanted 'an open, pokeable, companionable fire' and opposed the 'invasion of an Englishman's home'. In defence of 'liberty and property', they rejected ten attempted bills between 1884 and 1892. The onset of the First World War, and the subsequent housing crisis pushed concerns about air pollution into the background despite frequent smogs (Brimblecombe 1987; Ashby and Anderson 1981).

The first reports linking smoking with lung cancer and recommending that people stop smoking were hugely controversial. The *Express* presented itself as the defender of the ordinary smoker. It saw tobacco tax and advertising bans as a 'blow to freedom' and rejected health education pamphlets as government propaganda. *The Guardian*, in contrast, accepted people's freedom to smoke but supported government-sponsored public health campaigns (Hilton 2000).

Seatbelts caused furious controversy in parliamentary debates during the ten years before wearing them became mandatory in 1983. Some MPs saw their introduction as 'paternalism run rampant'; the act of a 'nanny state' restricting 'freedom of choice' for drivers. The role of law, they argued, was 'to protect the public at large and not the individual from his own harmful acts'. Others argued that individual freedom on the road was already constrained by innumerable regulations and that it was 'right for the state, with its knowledge and its power, to step in for the good of the community'. The law would not prevent people from driving, and so did not limit their freedom (Leichter 1986; House of Commons 1981–82).

Few people would now dispute the public and individual benefits of access to clean water, a sewerage system and clean air – these are infrastructural issues that individuals can do little on their own to create, but from which they benefit. And although alcohol, smoking and wearing a seatbelt appear to be 'personal' choices, few people would argue against the individual and social benefits of the legislation we now have in place.

Current debates

Today different issues command our attention: Should the government's ban on smoking in public places be partial or total? Should we ban junk food or have a fat tax or salt tax for processed food? Should we ban product advertising to children, or just control it? The issues are not just health related. The past few years have also seen debates ranging from whether the government should ban parents from smacking their children to whether teenagers wearing hoodies should be banned from shopping centres.

Since it came to power, the Labour government has been keen to distance itself from old-style big-government and avoid the nanny-statist label. It sees government as no longer 'intrusive' but 'enabling', and as 'doing things with people, not to them' (Fairclough 2000; *Daily Mail* 2001).

In *Choosing Health* it outlines government's protective role as one that 'strike[s] the right balance between allowing people to decide their own actions while not allowing those actions to unduly inconvenience or damage the health of others'. It sees its role as providing information, so individuals can make 'informed choices', providing personalised services to support motivated individuals, and facilitating partnerships with stakeholders, including industry, to encourage corporate responsibility. It believes this reflects a middle road between 'a paternalistic state' that 'limit[s] individual choice,... and ban[s]... unhealthy behaviour' and 'stand[ing] back, leaving people's health to whatever the hidden hand of the market and freedom of choice produces' (Department of Health 2004).

The Wanless report (2004) similarly believes there is a significant role for government in public health. It notes that 'individuals are ultimately responsible for their own and their children's health', but that government 'has a responsibility... to judge whether and to what extent it should intervene... to improve social welfare and population health'. It recognises that individuals do not always behave rationally, and this makes it legitimate for government to try 'shifting social norms' using regulations, taxes and subsidies as well as health services and information. Restrictive measures are acceptable, suggests Wanless, when they are 'justifiable in the public interest and to individuals as a reasonable restriction of their freedom'.

Media debates over where to draw the line between government intervention and individual responsibility take a more colourful, rhetorical approach. Some commentators support government intervention believing that it is justifiable in the public interest. They point out that individual choices often have costs for others, whether it be accidents caused by drunken driving, lung disease caused by passive smoking, or the costs of health care borne by tax-payers. Control over these issues lies beyond the power of any individual, but is within the ambit of the state. Others suggest that the state's 'duty' is 'to make it possible' for 'us to take more responsibility for our own health', by providing a health-promoting infrastructure, such as safe cycling routes, or school playing fields, and tackling poverty that gives rise to many lifestyle diseases (*The Guardian*, editorial 2004). Others favour stronger government regulations on food labelling, believing that this 'would allow people to take back control of their diet' and exercise their 'personal responsibility' as they have better information (Liberal Democrats 2004; Kennedy 2003).

Libertarian critics of government intervention respond with rallying calls for protecting individual freedom. They believe that individuals, not government, should decide whether and how much to smoke, drink, or eat and that those who advocate state curbs are, as one columnist put it, 'the forces of darkness: opposed to freedom, opposed to choice, and opposed to individual responsibility' (Pollard 2003). Forest, a tobacco-funded smokers' rights group, argues that 'it is up to individuals how they live their lives' and the 'right' to smoke or 'eat what you like', 'is as fundamental a freedom as the right to a free and private vote in elections' (Taylor and Fraser 2002). Some libertarians regard even government advice about healthier lifestyles as an unnecessary intrusion into personal lives, with some journalists describing it as 'relentless interference' and as 'propaganda' turning Britons 'into lifestyle automatons' (Starr 2004; Bristow 2004).

For libertarians, individuals are rational actors, who assess their choices in terms of cost and benefits to themselves and the state should not restrict this. As a columnist remarked, the 'right to take risks is an essential aspect of real freedom', despite the possible resulting harm (Luckhurst 2004). Other commentators are willing to balance individual liberties with the need for law to protect the collective from the individual, suggesting that 'adults must be allowed to harm themselves, but not others' (Glover 2004).

The public view

The conflicting media opinions about whether government should try to shape individuals' behaviour are matched by equal public confusion. The public is torn between believing that government has a role in improving and protecting public health, and reluctance to accept new interventions.

At one extreme, an opinion poll in 2005 identifies a significant segment of the population that supports curbs on private behaviour and accepts bans on chocolate machines in schools and hospitals, police cautions for pregnant women who smoke and bans on four-wheel drives in city centres (Future Foundation 2005).

Less extreme are the findings of a public opinion poll commissioned by the King's Fund (2004) which showed that most people believe that, while they do have responsibility for their own health, the government should improve health by providing information and advice, preventing actions that put the health of others at risk, and discouraging people from putting their own health at risk. However, poorer socio-economic groups are more likely to feel that health is beyond an individual's control and that tackling poverty is the most effective way for a government to prevent illness.

Analysis of other studies of public opinion on specific policies, such as alcohol, smoking and road safety, shows that people do not favour policies that limit their personal choices and view their own behaviour as benign, but they strongly favour stricter legislation controlling the potentially dangerous behaviour of others.

For example, there is little public support for measures that might affect people's access to alcohol. A Scottish survey found that just 1 per cent of respondents wanted to make alcohol more expensive, and 1 per cent wanted to ban 'happy hours' and other drink promotions, even though 86 per cent thought they led to increased drunkenness, binge drinking, crime and disorder (Scottish Executive Social Research 2003).

A survey commissioned by the Portman Group, an organisation set up by the drinks industry, showed that 80 per cent of respondents favoured a stricter drink-drive limit, a finding supported by other surveys. Yet only 13 per cent could identify the limit correctly and only a third could identify the number of units in any particular drink, suggesting that they did not feel a stricter limit would affect them personally (The Portman Group 2001; Quimby and Downing 1991; Lennox and Quimby 1990). Similarly, there was strong support in this survey for controls or a ban on TV and cinema advertising. However 87 per cent of respondents felt that advertising did not affect their own drinking, but 66 per cent felt it affected the drinking habits of other people (The Portman Group 2001).

Summary

The nanny-state debate is not new. Tensions between those favouring an interventionist state to promote the public interest and libertarians preferring a minimal state to ensure individual freedom, weave through the history of public health. Today, critics use the term 'nanny statist' to dismiss government measures believed to be too interventionist. In effect they are arguing over where we should draw the line between government and individual responsibility for health, and the principles that should guide government interventions.

What is often absent from the debate is an assessment of the possible benefits of state intervention, and an acknowledgement that the debate itself, is part of the process of changing attitudes and creating consensus about where to draw the line.

Ideas and attitudes change, and today it is doubtful that anyone would see laws ensuring we have a clean water supply and a sewerage system as a sign of excessive government, or a curb on civil liberties. We are unlikely to support the right of children to drink or smoke.

Restrictions on smoking are welcomed by many and people fasten their seatbelts with very little concern about its impact on their liberty. People recognise that restricting their freedom a little, allows them to live in greater safety and comfort and prevents harm to others. They recognise there are potential benefits for the individual and society in accepting laws that impinge a little on an individual's freedom.

Part 2 presents case studies on drinking, smoking and road safety. These draw on historical and contemporary evidence to assess the impact of encouraging, enabling and restrictive measures on general health and on the health of poorer socio-economic groups.

Part 2: Assessing the evidence

As discussed in Part 1, legislation, taxation and education are instruments that shape individual choices and create a safer public health framework. In this section, we examine how these have been applied, over time, to alcohol, smoking and road safety issues, such as seatbelts and drink-driving. Each case study begins with a summary of health impacts and costs, then sets out the interventions the government has taken at various points, and assesses their impact.

Alcohol

The health impact of alcohol

Moderate drinking reduces the risk of coronary heart disease and stroke for individuals, but at a population level there is a direct link between the quantity of alcohol consumed and the number of adults who die early (Babor, Caetano *et al* 2003).

Drinking contributes to morbidity (sickness) and mortality (deaths) from a range of cancers, cardiovascular conditions, neuropsychiatric conditions, such as alcohol dependence syndrome, gastro-intestinal conditions, such as liver cirrhosis, alcohol poisoning, low birth weight in babies and the retarded development of newborns. It is also linked with traffic accidents, occupational injuries, assaults and suicide.

ALCOHOL CONSUMPTION

In 1960, the per capita consumption of beer, wine, cider and spirits in Britain was 120 litres a year. This had risen to 170 litres by 2002 (Tighe 2003), although the average weekly consumption of alcohol in England is below government guidelines of three to four units a day for men (21 units a week) and two to three units a day for women (14 units a week) (Department of Health and Office for National Statistics 2004).

However, significant segments of the population drink above these limits, and women, 16 to 24 year olds, and teenagers are all now drinking more. In 2004, 27 per cent of men drank more than the recommended levels, as did 17 per cent of women – up from 12 per cent in 1992 (Department of Health and Office for National Statistics 2004).

Binge drinking is also a problem, with 21 per cent of men drinking more than eight units at once and 9 per cent of women drinking more than six units at once in a week. Among 16 to 24 year olds, the figures are even higher, with 34 per cent of young men, and 26 per cent of young women bingeing at least once a week (Department of Health and Office for National Statistics 2004).

More than a third of 15 year olds report having been drunk at age 13 or younger, compared to one in ten French or Italian children, and the amount they consume has risen from 5.3 units a week in 1990 to 10.5 in 2002 (Cabinet Office 2004).

ALCOHOL-RELATED COSTS

Alcohol-related morbidity and mortality is rising. NHS hospitals admitted 90,900 patients with a primary or secondary diagnosis of mental and behavioural disorders due to alcohol in 2002/03. They admitted 28,000 people for alcohol liver disease, double the number admitted in 1995/96 (Department of Health and Office for National Statistics 2004).

The total number of deaths directly related to alcohol has more than doubled from 2,506 in 1979 to 5,543 in 2000, of which 85 per cent were due to chronic liver disease and cirrhosis (Baker and Rooney 2003). Adding deaths due directly and indirectly to alcohol, brings the total to about 22,000 people dying prematurely each year (Cabinet Office Strategy Unit 2003).

The cost of alcohol misuse in England is about £20 billion a year. The NHS spends about £1.7 billion a year on alcohol-related cases, which account for two million bed days and a third of accident and emergency (A&E) attendances. Billions of pounds are also spent in dealing with alcohol-related crime and anti-social behaviour, or lost to the economy through ill health and trauma (*see* Figure 1) (Cabinet Office Strategy Unit 2003; Department of Health and Office for National Statistics 2004).

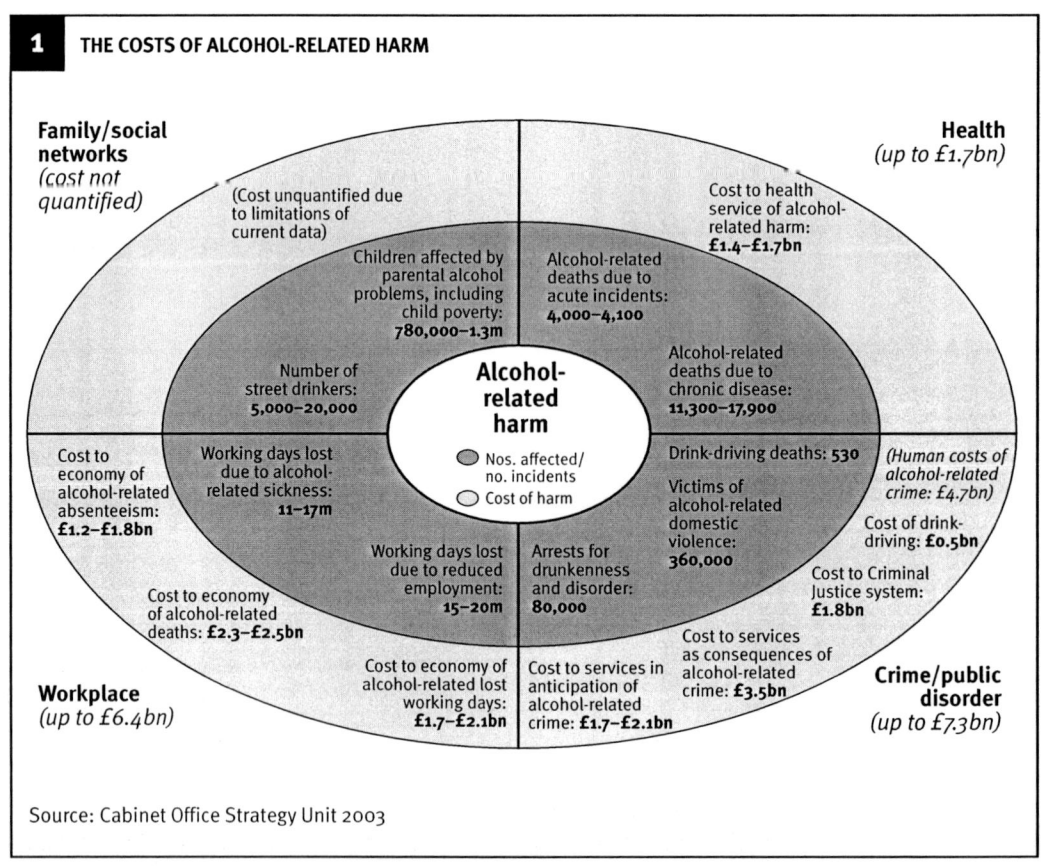

1 THE COSTS OF ALCOHOL-RELATED HARM

Source: Cabinet Office Strategy Unit 2003

Alcohol and health inequality

Consumption, morbidity and mortality also have a socio-economic dimension (*see* Figure 2). Consumption is highest in the highest and lowest socio-economic groups, although the latter also has higher levels of abstention than other social groups.

The lowest socio-economic groups are most likely to suffer alcohol dependence and alcohol-related mortality. Men aged 25–39 in class V (unskilled) are between ten and 20 times more likely to die from alcohol-related conditions than those in class I (professional). Men aged 55–64 in class V are two and a half to four times more likely to die than those in class I (Harrison and Gardiner 1999; Marmot and Feeney 1999; Whitehead 1987).

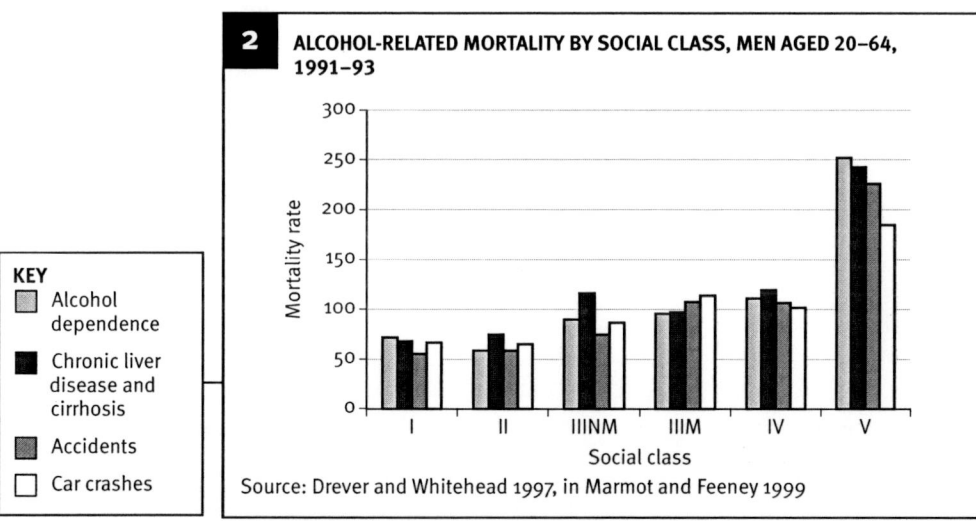

2 ALCOHOL-RELATED MORTALITY BY SOCIAL CLASS, MEN AGED 20–64, 1991–93

KEY
- Alcohol dependence
- Chronic liver disease and cirrhosis
- Accidents
- Car crashes

Source: Drever and Whitehead 1997, in Marmot and Feeney 1999

History

In the early 1800s, public drunkenness was acceptable, with children drinking as freely as adults. Just over a century later, alcohol consumption had dropped dramatically and it was no longer acceptable for children to drink. There were cultural and legislative changes that brought this about.

The temperance movement gradually changed attitudes to alcohol and public drunkenness, and created alternative leisure activities to the pub. From the 1830s, an evangelical temperance movement began to preach to working men, persuading them to improve themselves through abstention, self-education and thrift. By the 1850s, a rival prohibitionist movement began to focus on parliamentary reform to regulate the drink trade (Harrison 1971).

The temperance movement expanded until there were temperance-friendly societies, life assurance companies offering sober clientele better terms, temperance hotels and coffee houses. Thomas Cook, a temperance propagandist and travelling preacher, chartered the first temperance excursions as an alternative to drunken revels on workers' holidays.

As city administrators took over urban water supplies, water quality improved and drinking water was made available in poorer parts of cities. Tea duty declined and tea became cheaper than beer for the poor. Ginger beer, lemonade and soda water were new drinks that gradually became available in pubs. It became gentlemanly to remain sober, especially among the well-to-do.

Government legislation controlling the sale of alcohol also played a role in changing consumption habits. A key piece of legislation was the Licensing Act in 1872, which restricted opening hours for pubs from 5am to midnight on weekdays, and 1pm to 11pm on Sundays, with a two-hour afternoon break. It also prohibited children from drinking spirits in a pub, and later from buying spirits to take away; and increased penalties for drunken behaviour. The number of pubs began to decline, as did the consumption of beer and spirits, albeit very slowly (Burnett 1999; Harrison 1971).

Of far greater impact, however, was stringent government action during the First World War. The government used its emergency powers to control the drink trade. Beer duty trebled between 1914 and 1918, and its price more than doubled, while the price of spirits trebled. The government reduced pub opening hours from 17 hours a day to just five and a half, regulated the strength of alcohol, diverted home-grown grain from drink to food manufacture, and portrayed heavy drinking as unpatriotic. After the war, controls were relaxed but opening hours were kept shorter, and the sale of drinks to under-18s was finally prohibited in 1923.

The harsh legislation was also complemented by social changes that encouraged sobriety. There were new places to socialise, such as the cinema, tea shops and corner houses such as Lyons, while milk bars became popular from the late 1920s – as radio began to keep men at home in the evenings. Malted milk drinks, such as Ovaltine, Bournvita and Horlicks, were intensively advertised to adults.

By 1932, a Royal Commission on Licensing noted that 'drunkenness has gone out of fashion and a drunken person is not tolerated as he used to be' (cited in Rose 1984). And faced with a declining market, the drinks industry complained that 'millions of young men' did not have 'the beer drinking habit instilled'. In 1901, people drank on average 135 litres of beer and 4.5 litres of spirits. By 1935, this had dropped to 60 litres of beer and 0.9 litres of spirits.

Alcohol consumption and alcohol-related deaths only began to rise again in the post-war period (Plant 1997; Baker and Rooney 2003). The introduction of commercial television in the 1950s gave the industry a platform from which to glamorise drinking for a huge audience. At the same time licensing laws began to be liberalised, working-class incomes increased and the price of alcohol began to decline (International Study of Alcohol Control Experiences and World Health Organisation Regional Office for Europe 1981).

The reversal of earlier government policy since the 1950s has also increased inequalities. In the 1950s, alcohol consumption and mortality were highest in social class I, since people in this group could afford to drink to excess. By the 1980s, alcohol-related mortality was higher in class V (Harrison and Gardiner 1999; Marmot and Feeney 1999).

Effective interventions

This review of the UK experience over the past 150 years suggests that alcohol consumption and the problems related to it have fallen when the sale of alcohol has been restricted, and it has been heavily taxed. But shifts in cultural attitudes and behaviour were also important. Sobriety became socially acceptable, and the temperance movement helped create opportunities for new products, markets and leisure activities as alternatives to alcohol.

The following section looks in more detail at research findings on the effectiveness of taxation, licensing, restrictions on advertising and health education as ways for governments to control the impact of alcohol on public health.

TAXATION

International studies show that increasing the price of alcohol generally leads to a decrease in consumption, with a positive follow-on effect for public health. In the United Kingdom, alcohol consumption has increased as the price of alcohol relative to income has fallen (*see* Figure 3). Since 1980, beer taxes have stayed constant in real terms (that is, after adjusting for inflation), but tax on wine and spirits – where consumption has been rising – have fallen in real terms. Households' disposable income has also increased by 91 per cent over the past 20 years, making alcohol more affordable (Department of Health and Office for National Statistics 2004).

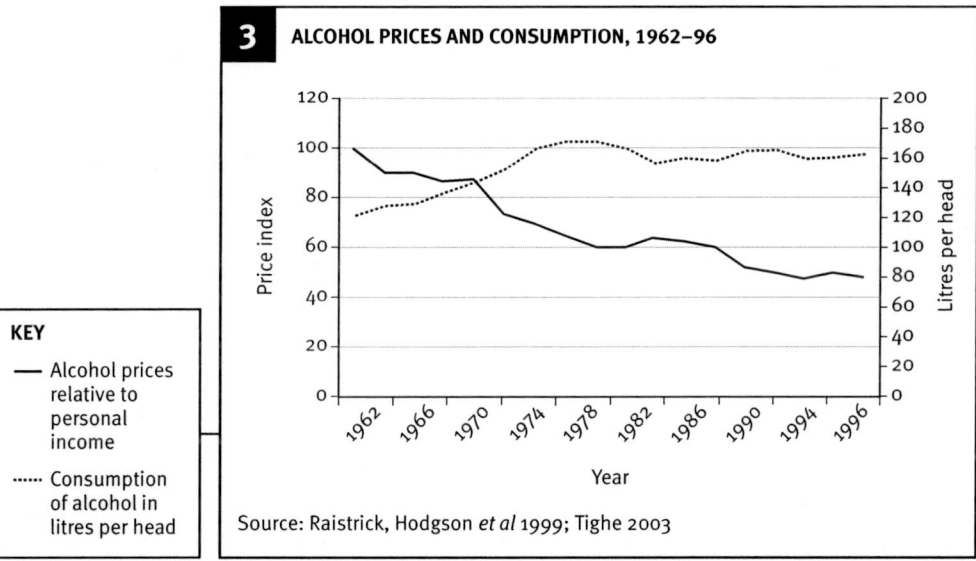

3 **ALCOHOL PRICES AND CONSUMPTION, 1962–96**

KEY
— Alcohol prices relative to personal income
····· Consumption of alcohol in litres per head

Source: Raistrick, Hodgson *et al* 1999; Tighe 2003

Countries that increase the price of alcohol through tax find that consumption decreases. In 1992, the Northern Territory in Australia introduced a harm reduction levy on all drinks with over 3 per cent alcohol. Over the four following years, per capita consumption decreased by 22 per cent and alcohol-related morbidity and mortality also declined (Crosbie, Stockwell *et al* 2000).

US studies have found that states with higher alcohol taxes have fewer deaths from liver cirrhosis, fewer motor vehicle fatalities, especially among young adults, and fewer homicides, rapes, robberies, assaults, motor vehicle thefts and cases of domestic violence and child abuse (Edwards, Anderson *et al* 1994; Chaloupka, Grossman *et al* 2002).

There are no consistent findings on the impact of tax and price increases on the drinking patterns of heavy drinkers, some of whom will come from the poorer socio-economic groups (Godfrey 1997). Heavy drinkers appear more likely to switch to another type of alcohol when one is more strongly taxed (Waller, Naidoo *et al* 2002). Targeting taxation at young people is also difficult, as drinking fashions change quickly (Waller, Naidoo *et al* 2002).

RESTRICTING AVAILABILITY

Completely banning access to alcohol would be politically unacceptable, and would most likely encourage illegal drinking (and, if the US experience of 'prohibition' is anything to go by, crime). However, restricting access to alcohol seems to reduce consumption rates.

When Sweden allowed its liquor stores to open on Saturday, sales of alcohol increased, but so did rates of domestic violence and public drunkenness. The Saturday closure was reinstituted (Olsson and Wikstrom 1982).

When Scotland relaxed its licensing hours in 1976, alcohol consumption increased by 13 per cent, even though it remained unchanged in the rest of the United Kingdom, where hours remained the same. However, when England and Wales relaxed their opening hours in 1988, only consumption by heavy drinkers appeared to increase (Raistrick, Hodgson *et al* 1999).

ADVERTISING BANS

There is conflicting evidence about the extent to which advertising influences alcohol consumption.

A study that compared 17 countries over a 13-year period found that those with total bans on beer, wine and spirits advertising had lower alcohol consumption levels, lower mortality due to cirrhosis of the liver and fewer motor vehicle fatalities than countries that only banned spirit advertising or allowed advertising. A follow-up study with data from 20 countries spanning a 26-year period, similarly found that banning alcohol advertising resulted in a decrease in consumption (Saffer 1991). However, studies in Britain, Canada and the United States in the 1980s suggested that advertising has little impact on the total consumption of alcohol, although it might affect the demand for particular drinks or brands. Critics suggest this is because the media market is so heavily saturated. They also say the real impact of advertising is in the way that it shapes attitudes to drinking (Babor, Caetano *et al* 2003). US studies of teenagers and college students show that repeated exposure to adverts cultivated views of 'typical' drinkers as fun-loving, happy and good-looking and this was associated with more favourable attitudes to drinking.

A New Zealand study of young people found that participants who gave a more positive response to alcohol advertising at 18 were heavier drinkers and reported more alcohol-related aggression at age 21, a finding repeated when the same group of youngsters was re-interviewed at the age of 26 (Casswell, Pledger *et al* 2002; Casswell and Zhang 1998).

EDUCATION

Health awareness programmes aim to change individuals' knowledge and attitudes about risks related to drinking, in the hope that this will affect behaviour. The evidence is that mass-media campaigns are cost effective, because they reach a high percentage of their target audience, but that they have only some impact on knowledge and attitudes and little impact on behaviour (Raistrick, Hodgson *et al* 1999).

Evaluations of warning labels (used in the United States to highlight the risks of drinking while pregnant or when driving) show that labels make drinkers more aware of the risks, but do not change their behaviour, and that labels can make alcohol more attractive to teenagers and young adults (Babor, Caetano 2003).

In Britain, health promotion campaigns are least noticed by men, under-25s and people from lower income groups IV and V, that is, the groups most likely to drink heavily (The Portman Group 2001). One survey showed that men, under-25s and respondents from classes IV and V were most likely to say that they were more likely to disregard health promotion campaigns.

School education programmes have shifted from an informative and factual approach about the effects of alcohol misuse, to models that also teach social skills needed to deal with everyday stresses. Evaluations of school-based information and normative programmes show they have at best, short-lived, modest effects, and do not delay the onset of drinking nor sustain reduced drinking, and do not prevent alcohol misuse. A review of school-based education and normative programmes concludes that they 'cannot be supported as a major plank of a prevention policy' (Raistrick, Hodgson *et al* 1999; Babor, Caetano 2003).

Summary

The story of government action on alcohol is one of increasingly stringent restrictions followed by liberalisation. Historical and contemporary research suggests that strong state action is effective in limiting people's access to alcohol and the volume they drink and that this has a positive effect on their health.

Alcohol consumption and related disease declines when governments increase alcohol taxes, restrict the availability of alcohol by controlling the density of outlets, sales hours or pub-opening times, and ban advertising. Both consumption and alcohol-related problems increase when prices fall relative to real incomes, taxes drop, and access is liberalised. Education programmes raise awareness but do not change behaviour.

However, the historical evidence also shows that cultural change is important. The 19th-century temperance movement and the new industries that sprang up to cater to more sober tastes also helped to change cultural attitudes to drinking and offered alternatives to the pub. It is evident that attitudes to drinking have changed in the post-war era too, as alcohol has become more accessible, and public drunkenness and bingeing more socially acceptable in some groups. But public concern about the impact of 24-hour licensing on drunkenness and violence suggests that the limits of acceptability may have been reached.

Smoking

The health impact of smoking

Smoking-related diseases include lung cancer, chronic lung disease, such as bronchitis and emphysema, and coronary heart disease. Smokers also face a higher risk than non-smokers of cancers of the mouth, throat, oesophagus, larynx, pancreas, bladder and cervix.

Passive smoking increases the risk of bronchitis, pneumonia, asthma, cot death and possibly of cardiovascular and neurobiological impairment in children. One in two long-term smokers dies prematurely as a result of smoking, and half of these deaths occur in middle age (Action on Smoking and Health (ASH) 2004a).

PREVALENCE

In 1950, an estimated 65 per cent of men and 40 per cent of women smoked in the United Kingdom. Today, about 27 per cent of the adult population smokes (14 million people) (*see* Figure 4). However, smoking is on the increase among children aged 11 to 15 in England. In 1988, 8 per cent of this age group smoked regularly. By 1996, it was 13 per cent (Department of Health 1998b).

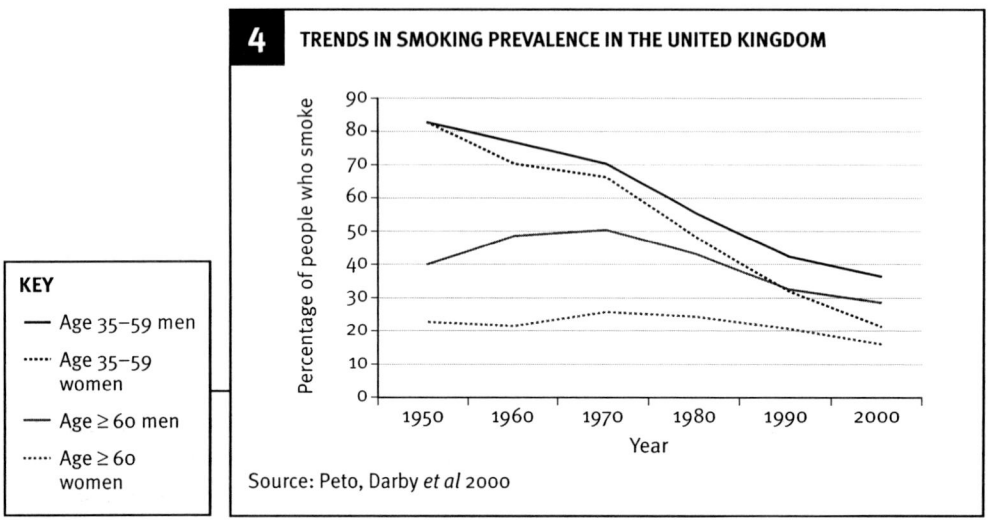

KEY
— Age 35–59 men
····· Age 35–59 women
— Age ≥ 60 men
····· Age ≥ 60 women

4 TRENDS IN SMOKING PREVALENCE IN THE UNITED KINGDOM

Source: Peto, Darby *et al* 2000

THE COSTS OF SMOKING

In 1965, 106,000 men in the United Kingdom died due to tobacco-related illnesses – 32.8 per cent of all male deaths. By 2000, it was down to 63,000 – 21.7 per cent of all male deaths (*see* Figure 5, opposite) (Peto, Lopez *et al* 2004).

Female mortality due to smoking has risen over the same period, because women took up smoking later than men. In 1965, 17,000 women in the United Kingdom died due to tobacco-related illnesses – 5.6 per cent of all female deaths. By 1995, it was up to 51,000 – 16 per cent of all female deaths (Peto, Lopez *et al* 2004). Women under 65 in the United Kingdom have the worst death rate from lung cancer of all EU countries except Denmark (Department of Health 1998a).

Smoking-related diseases still cause about 120,000 deaths a year – about one-fifth of annual deaths in the United Kingdom (Department of Health 2003). Smoking costs the NHS approximately £1.5 billion a year, and also carries an economic cost. It is estimated that 34 million working days are lost to British industry every year from smoking-related sick leave (ASH 2004a).

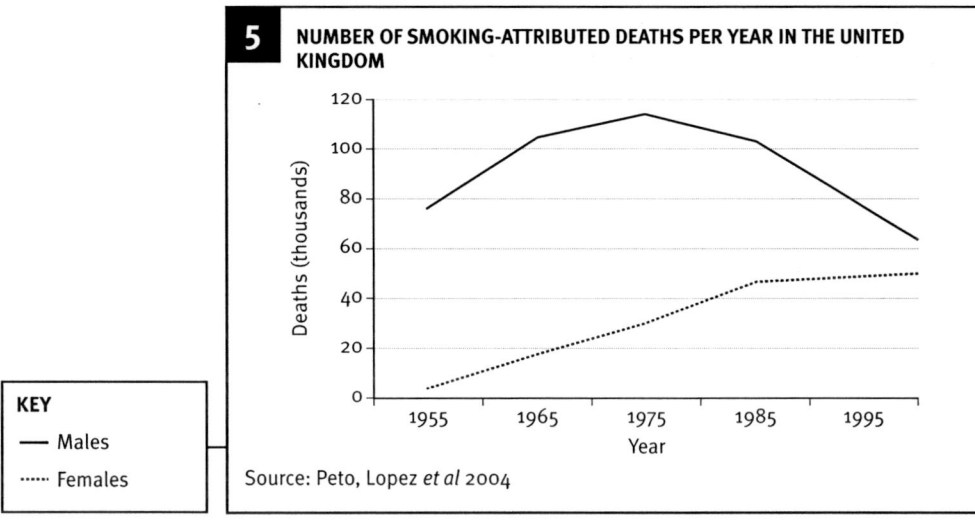

5 NUMBER OF SMOKING-ATTRIBUTED DEATHS PER YEAR IN THE UNITED KINGDOM

Source: Peto, Lopez *et al* 2004

KEY
— Males
······ Females

SMOKING AND INEQUALITIES

The downwards trend in smoking and mortality has a socio-economic dimension; it is largely the middle classes who have changed their habits. Between 1973 and 1996, smoking cessation rates increased from 25 per cent to over 50 per cent in higher income groups, but from 8–9 per cent to 10–13 per cent in poorer groups (Acheson 1998, in Richardson 2001).

In 2001, 34 per cent of those in manual occupations smoked, compared to 15 per cent of higher managers and professionals (Department of Health 2003). In the most deprived groups, smoking prevalence reaches over 70 per cent, and among homeless people sleeping rough, about 90 per cent (Health Development Agency and ASH 2001).

Higher rates of smoking translate into higher rates of illness and mortality (*see* Figure 6, p 18). It is estimated that half the difference in survival to 70 years between social classes I and V is due to higher smoking prevalence in class V (Department of Health analysis quoted in Wanless 2004).

There is relatively little research to assess what works for lower socio-economic groups (Naidoo, Warm *et al* 2004). The high rates of smoking among those who can least afford it are due to a combination of social and personal factors, ranging from the social environment and parental models, to economic insecurity, isolation, stress and feelings of hopelessness (Richardson 2001). People in disadvantaged groups are just as likely to want to quit as others, but enabling factors, such as changes in employment opportunities or optimism about the future, are far less common. They also have low health expectations and find it hard to feel positive about their future health (Jarvis, Wardle *et al* 2003; Richardson 2001) (*see* Figure 7, p 18).

History

In 1883, a Bristol tobacco manufacturer bought sole rights to a cigarette-making machine. This transformed the industry in Britain. Previously, tobacco products had been luxury, hand-made items. Now they became a cheap, mass-produced commodity, and by the end of the First World War, cigarettes dominated the tobacco market (Hilton 2000).

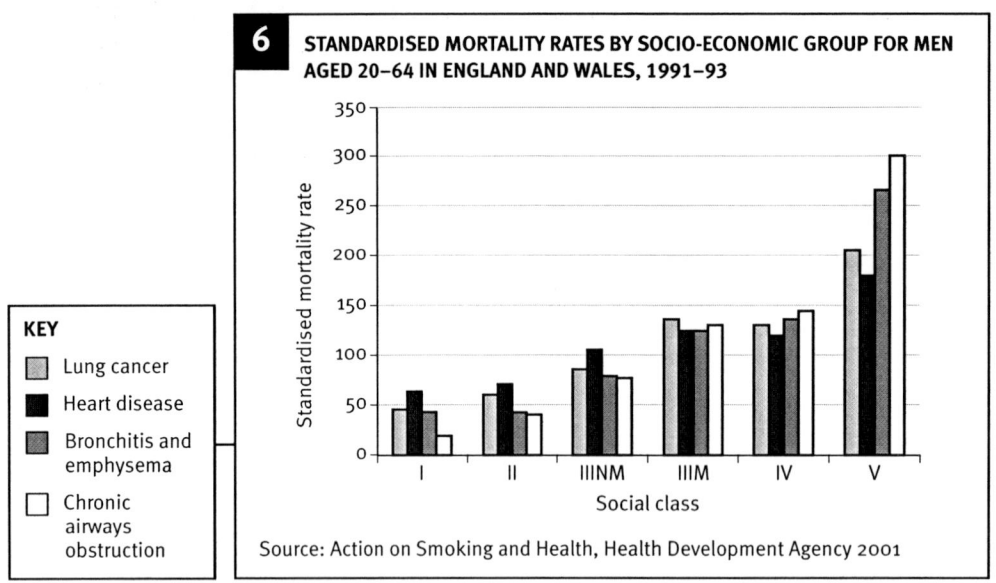

6 **STANDARDISED MORTALITY RATES BY SOCIO-ECONOMIC GROUP FOR MEN AGED 20–64 IN ENGLAND AND WALES, 1991–93**

KEY
- Lung cancer
- Heart disease
- Bronchitis and emphysema
- Chronic airways obstruction

Source: Action on Smoking and Health, Health Development Agency 2001

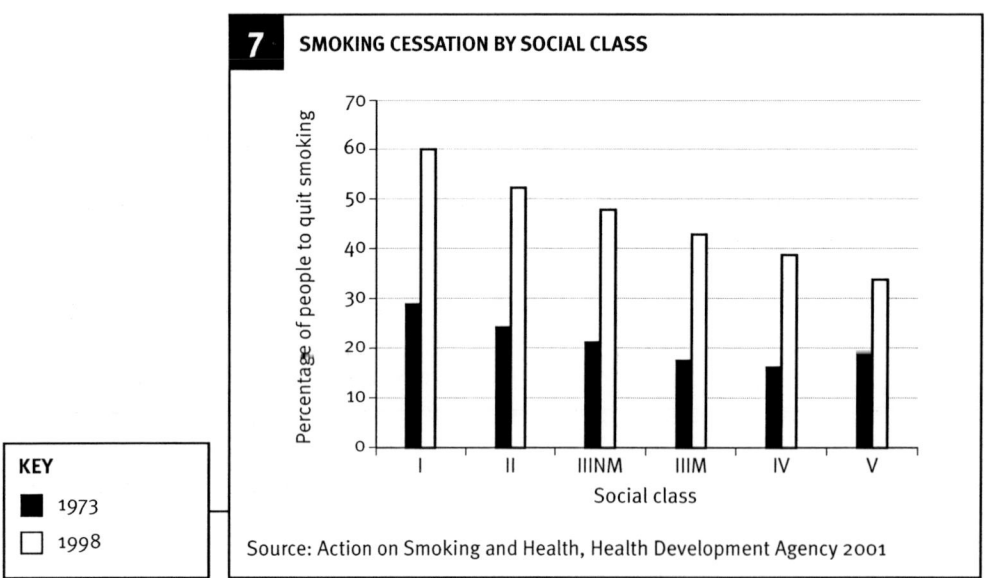

7 **SMOKING CESSATION BY SOCIAL CLASS**

KEY
- 1973
- 1998

Source: Action on Smoking and Health, Health Development Agency 2001

The same period saw the rapid growth of the popular press following the abolition of various taxes. New consumer magazines appeared and manufacturers used the burgeoning advertising market to shape consumer demands.

As with the history of alcohol, controls over smoking have been a result of cultural and political changes. A popular anti-smoking movement was slow to emerge. The first Anti-Tobacco Society was set up in the early 1850s, but never attracted much public enthusiasm and remained on the fringes of the temperance movement (*see* p 11). The Children's Act of 1908 was the first legislation to regulate access to tobacco, and made it an offence to sell tobacco to a child under 16. It was the result of a campaign led by children's welfare reformers, and reflected new, idealised notions about childhood, and fears about declining national vigour, rather than the beginnings of a widespread popular anti-smoking movement.

Far more significant in shaping cultural attitudes against smoking has been the medical evidence about the connection between smoking and ill health. Richard Doll and Austin Bradford Hill published the first epidemiological evidence of a link between tobacco and lung cancer in 1950. Their work was complemented by a similar study in the United States later the same year. At the time, some medical and scientific experts dismissed the statistical correlations because carcinogenic agents had not yet been found in tobacco, and others believed that air pollution was a more likely cause (Hilton 2000; Berridge 1998).

Throughout the 1950s, the attitude of the Ministry of Health was one of complacency and denial. Despite mounting scientific evidence, the Ministry initially refused to consider anti-smoking campaigns or a ban on cigarette advertising because it felt further proof was still needed. It believed that it was up to individuals to weigh up the evidence and risks and act as they saw fit, rather than for government to intervene. The Health Minister chain-smoked his way through the first, cautious government statement on cancer and smoking in 1954 (Pollock 1992). The complacency was also fostered by close links with the tobacco industry, which the industry continued to cultivate throughout the 1970s and 1980s (Pollock 1992; Taylor 1984).

Action on Smoking and Health (ASH), an anti-smoking group, was set up in 1971 with funding from the Department of Health and Social Security. It lobbied to raise tobacco tax, ban sports sponsorships, and restrict advertising. It also worked with a range of voluntary-sector organisations, such as the British Heart Foundation and the Cancer Research Campaign, on anti-smoking public education messages. In reaction, the tobacco industry set up and funded Forest in 1979, to defend 'freedom of choice' and 'liberty'. Smoking controls became politically controversial and newspapers debated the acceptable extent of state intervention (Hilton 2000).

Despite its reluctant start, the government slowly began to introduce fiscal, regulatory and voluntary controls to discourage smoking. The United Kingdom now has the highest priced cigarettes in the European Union and one of the highest levels of duty on cigarettes in the world (Wanless 2004). Almost 80 per cent of the price of a packet of cigarettes consists of taxation, earning the government £9.6 billion in revenue from tobacco in 2000 (ASH 2002). In recent years, the UK government has raised tobacco duty in each budget in line with inflation.

Until 1965, the government relied on a voluntary advertising code on television. It then banned cigarette advertising on television, and later extended the ban to cinema and radio. In 2003, as a signatory to the World Health Organisation (WHO) Framework Convention on Tobacco Control, it finally prohibited tobacco advertising across all media, and ended tobacco promotion and sponsorship of events.

The government has also introduced warning labels on cigarette packaging. Under the WHO convention, these must cover at least 30 per cent (and preferably 50 per cent) of cigarette packaging, and misleading tobacco product descriptors such as 'light' and 'mild' are prohibited (ASH 2004c).

In the past 20 years, the UK government has relied on voluntary action by employers and industry to curb smoking in public places. Cinema chains, airlines, hospitals, post offices, transport providers and local government have all introduced voluntary smoking restrictions.

However, 52 per cent of workplaces are still not smoke free (Fichtenberg and Glantz 2002), 46 per cent of restaurants and bars still allow smoking and only 22 per cent provide separate smoking and non-smoking areas (ASH 2004b).

In 2004, the government decided not to ban smoking in all public places. Instead, all enclosed public places and workplaces (including government departments and NHS buildings) and licensed premises serving food will be smoke free, and pubs and bars will be free to choose (Department of Health 2004).

Effective interventions

In the past hundred years, smoking has moved from an unregulated to a restricted activity, and the result has been beneficial for public health. The following section looks at contemporary international and UK evidence on the health impact of taxation, advertising bans, restrictions on smoking in public places, and education campaigns.

TAXATION

A World Bank and WHO study on the economics of tobacco control found tax increases 'the single most effective intervention to reduce the demand for tobacco' in low- and middle- income countries. The study concluded that raising the real price of cigarettes by 10 per cent reduced smoking by about 8 per cent (Jha and Chaloupka 2000). It also concluded that price increases induce some smokers to quit and prevent others from becoming regular or persistent smokers. Children and adolescents are more responsive to changes in the price of consumer goods than adults, and if the price goes up, they are more likely to reduce their consumption (World Bank 2001).

These findings are confirmed by studies in high-income countries such as the United States and United Kingdom (Melihan-Cheinin and Hirsch 1997). When Massachusetts imposed substantial tax increases on cigarettes in 1993, consumption fell by 4 per cent compared to a 1 per cent decrease in other states that had not introduced the tax (Biener, Harris *et al* 2000).

A UK study shows that as tobacco prices increased from the 1970s, consumption began to decline (*see* Figure 8, opposite). However, when tax failed to keep up with inflation, as happened between 1977 and 1979, smoking increased by 10 per cent (Townsend, Roderick *et al* 1994; Melihan-Cheinin and Hirsch 1997).

Another UK study showed that price changes had most effect on lower socio-economic groups, reducing the number of cigarettes smoked, and the number of smokers (Townsend *et al* 1994). New York recently introduced a ban on smoking in public places and an 18-fold increase in cigarette taxes. This too cut the number of adult smokers: from 2002 to 2003, the number of adult smokers in the city fell by 11 per cent, while smokers who did not quit smoked 13 per cent less. The fall in smokers occurred across all boroughs, ages, and ethnic groups but was most marked among the poorest, especially the young, ethnic minorities and women (Miller 2005).

However, tax-led price rises also have a disproportionate impact on the household income of poorer income groups. The poorest tenth of the population in the United Kingdom spends around 15 per cent of weekly income on cigarettes, compared to a national average of 2 per cent (Health Development Agency and ASH 2001). In the United Kingdom, cigarette smuggling now accounts for 18 per cent of the market, which reduces the effectiveness of taxation on consumption (Wanless 2004).

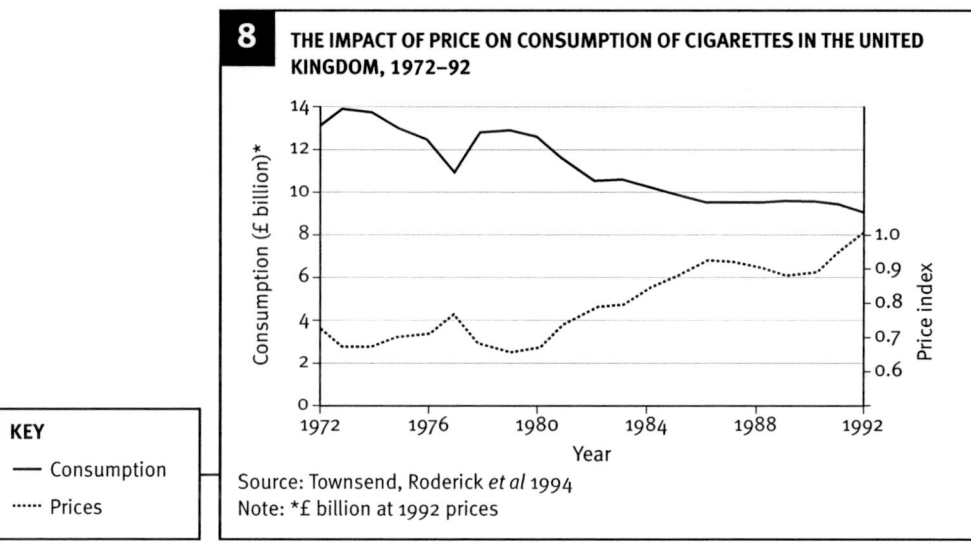

8 | **THE IMPACT OF PRICE ON CONSUMPTION OF CIGARETTES IN THE UNITED KINGDOM, 1972–92**

Source: Townsend, Roderick *et al* 1994
Note: *£ billion at 1992 prices

ADVERTISING

Advertising bans have a direct impact on consumption rates. A survey of advertising bans in 102 countries showed that partial bans have little or no effect, since tobacco companies switch to other media and to sponsorship, but comprehensive media bans reduce consumption (Saffer and Chaloupka 2000; ASH 2004d).

Norway, Finland and Iceland were among the first countries to ban tobacco advertising in the 1970s, and saw substantial reductions in smoking rates and tobacco consumption. In Iceland, smoking prevalence among 12–16 year olds dropped from 32 per cent in 1974 to 13 per cent in 1986, following a ban in 1971 (Melihan-Cheinin and Hirsch 1997).

The Department of Health estimates that banning tobacco advertising and promotion in the United Kingdom will result in a 2.5 per cent reduction in the number of deaths caused by smoking, eventually saving up to 3,000 lives a year (Department of Health 1998a).

RESTRICTING SMOKING IN PUBLIC SPACES

California banned smoking in all enclosed places of employment in 1995, New South Wales in Australia followed in 2000, New York in March 2003, and Ireland in March 2004. Scottish ministers plan to follow in 2006.

Compliance with such regulation depends on a widespread consensus among smokers and non-smokers about the ethics of public smoking, since regulations have to be enforced largely through peer pressure and social conformity, rather than financial or legal penalties (Jha and Chaloupka 2000).

Research shows that bans on smoking in public places have two effects. First, they reduce non-smokers' exposure to tobacco smoke. For example, a study of bartenders in San Francisco showed improvements in respiratory health within two months of implementing a ban on indoor smoking (Eisner, Smith *et al* 1998). A study of restaurant and bar workers in New York before and after the complete ban on smoking in public places was introduced showed reduced cotinine levels among non-smokers (cotinine is a nicotine by-product found in the body fluids of people who have inhaled tobacco smoke) and reduced self-reported respiratory symptoms (Farrelly, Nonnemaker *et al* 2005).

Second, 'clean air' policies reduce an individual's tobacco consumption and so encourage smokers to quit. A review of 26 studies of smoke-free workplaces in four countries concluded that totally smoke-free workplaces are twice as effective at reducing consumption and prevalence as policies that restrict smoking to a few designated areas. Total workplace bans result in a 3.8 per cent reduction in smoking prevalence, with each smoker consuming 3.1 fewer cigarettes per day (Fichtenberg and Glantz 2002).

It has been estimated that if the government was to introduce a workplace smoking ban across the United Kingdom, per capita cigarette consumption could decline by 7.6 per cent (Fichtenberg and Glantz 2002).

EDUCATION
More than 65 per cent of adult smokers across the socio-economic spectrum would like to quit smoking (ASH and Health Development Agency 2003). Smokers are also aware of the impact of passive smoking on the health of other people. In a recent poll, 68 per cent of smokers said they did not smoke at all when a child was in the room (up from 66 per cent in 2002) and 46 per cent said they would modify their smoking in the company of adult non-smokers (Office for National Statistics 2003).

These attitudes are likely to be the result of 30 years of campaigning by anti-smoking lobbyists, high taxation, advertising bans and limitations on smoking in public places, since the evidence for the impact of mass-media campaigns on attitudes and behaviour is equivocal.

Some research suggests that, as with alcohol-education programmes, awareness of the health risks of smoking does not equate with a change in behaviour. A review of international evidence showed that isolated anti-smoking programmes for teenagers at best delay the onset of smoking, but are unlikely to prevent it (Grey, Owen *et al* 2000; Health Development Agency 2004).

Studies of smokers' attitudes show that where individuals understand the links between smoking and ill health, they often associate cancer with those who are heavier smokers than themselves, or have ready examples of elderly relatives who smoked without harm until their deaths. They do not associate anti-smoking messages with themselves, but see them as useful for others and support solutions that remove responsibility from themselves (Hilton 2000).

Other research suggests that although it is difficult to assess the impact of mass-media campaigns because attitudes and behaviour change slowly, such campaigns can be associated with a decline in smoking when they are part of a comprehensive tobacco-control policy that also includes high taxation, advertising bans and bans on smoking in public places. Media campaigns show smokers that they are not alone, offer support and encouragement in ongoing attempts to quit, and provide clear reasons for quitting (Grey, Owen *et al* 2000; Richardson 2001). Smokers exposed to mass-media campaigns are also more likely to quit than those who are not (Naidoo, Warm *et al* 2004; Health Development

Agency 2004). Health promotion campaigns are most effective at reducing smoking in higher socio-economic groups (Townsend, Roderick *et al* 1994).

Summary

The history of government action on smoking is one of initially reluctant intervention and then gradually increasing willingness to shape the market and consumption patterns.

Historical and contemporary research suggests that strong government action has led to smokers smoking less and more people quitting. Mortality and morbidity from tobacco-related diseases have also fallen in recent decades. Tobacco consumption decreases when governments increase taxes, ban advertising and ban smoking in public places. Education programmes raise awareness, although their impact on behaviour is uncertain. However, education campaigns have certainly contributed to gradual cultural changes, with smokers less likely to smoke in front of children, or in the company of non-smokers, and increasing public support for a ban on smoking in public places.

Road safety: seatbelts and drink-driving

The health impact

Britain has the lowest deaths per capita per kilometre travelled in the world: 5.9 people out of every 100,000 inhabitants are killed on the roads each year in the United Kingdom, compared to 11 in every 100,000 in the European Union as a whole (Dyer 2004). Casualties peaked in the mid-1960s and since then have gradually fallen. In 1965, there were 405,952 deaths and injuries, while in 2003 there were 294,508, even though the number of vehicles had tripled (*see* Figure 9, p 24) (Department for Transport 2003c).

Prevalence

COSTS OF NOT WEARING A SEATBELT

In October 2004, 93 per cent of drivers, 94 per cent of front-seat passengers, 93 per cent of rear-seat child passengers, but only 65 per cent of rear-seat adult passengers wore seatbelts (Department for Transport 2004). Seatbelts reduce the risk of death or injury. An unbelted driver or passenger in a car that crashes at 30 mph will be thrown forward with a force 30 to 60 times his or her body weight. Each year 8 to 15 front-seat passengers are killed by unbelted rear-seat passengers. However, in 2001 wearing a seatbelt was estimated to have saved 2,278 lives and prevented 95,000 minor and 23,000 serious casualties (Department for Transport 2001).

COSTS OF DRINK-DRIVING

The number of people killed or seriously injured in drink-drive accidents in Britain has fallen from over 9,000 in the 1980s to less than 4,000 in the 1990s, and is now around 3,000. In 2002, 550 people died in drink-drive accidents, 2,790 were seriously injured and 16,760 were slightly injured. Male drivers under 25 are the most likely to be involved in a drink-driving accident. Drink-drive accidents account for 6 per cent of all road casualties and 16 per cent of road deaths (Mosedale, Francis *et al* 2003).

FINANCIAL COSTS

The direct cost of deaths and injuries from road accidents in the United Kingdom is estimated to be £3 billion a year (Department for Transport 2000). The total cost of medical treatment, loss of earnings, pain, suffering or loss of life, and vehicle damage is estimated to be £17.76 billion per year (Department for Transport 2003b).

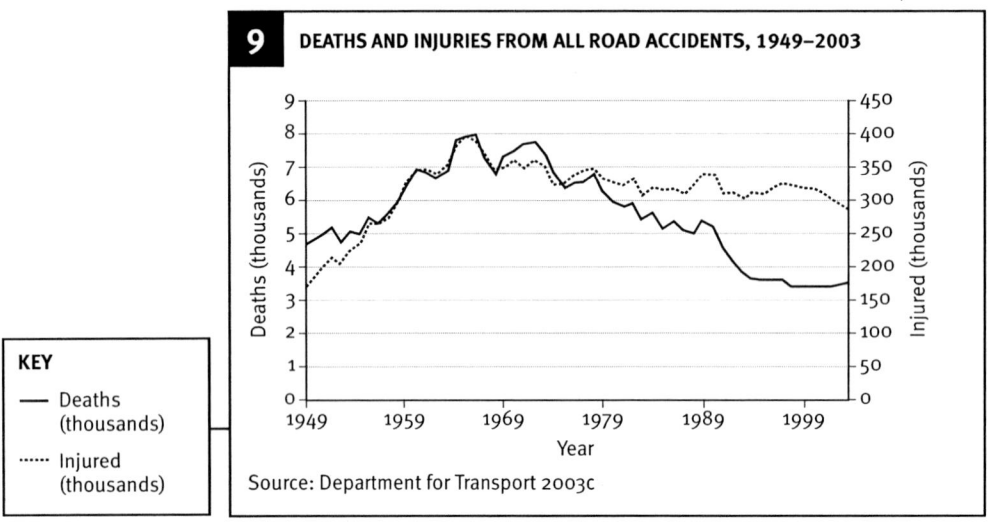

9 DEATHS AND INJURIES FROM ALL ROAD ACCIDENTS, 1949–2003

KEY

— Deaths (thousands)

····· Injured (thousands)

Source: Department for Transport 2003c

History

Today's low casualty and fatality rate from road accidents is due, in part, to laws making seatbelt use mandatory and making it illegal to drive while intoxicated.

Britain was one of the first countries to require front seatbelts to be fitted to cars in 1965. The first UK bill for mandatory seatbelt use was introduced in 1973, but failed, as did another six efforts over the following decade. The seventh attempt began as a Conservative Party Private Member's Bill in the House of Lords in 1980, which was opposed by the Secretary of State for Transport, the leaders of both parties and their Chief Whips, but eventually approved after a free vote (Leichter 1986; Mackay 1987; McCarthy 1989). The government finally made front-seatbelt use compulsory for drivers and front-seat passengers in 1983, rear-seatbelt use mandatory for children in 1989, and rear-seatbelt use for adults mandatory in 1991.

In the Road Safety Act of 1967, the government made it an offence to drive with a blood-alcohol concentration limit (BAC limit) above 0.8 grams per litre, introduced breathalyser testing, and permitted the police to breath-test drivers they suspect of drinking, committing a driving offence, or being involved in an accident. Drivers are disqualified for a minimum of a year if convicted of a drink-driving offence.

Effective interventions
MANDATORY SEATBELTS

Making seatbelts mandatory had an immediate impact on compliance. Between February 1982 and February 1983, seatbelt use jumped from 37 per cent to 93 per cent for drivers and from 39 per cent to 93 per cent for front-seat passengers. Between October 1990 and October 1991, rear-seatbelt use jumped from 43 per cent to 63 per cent (*see* Figure 10, opposite) (Department of Transport 2004).

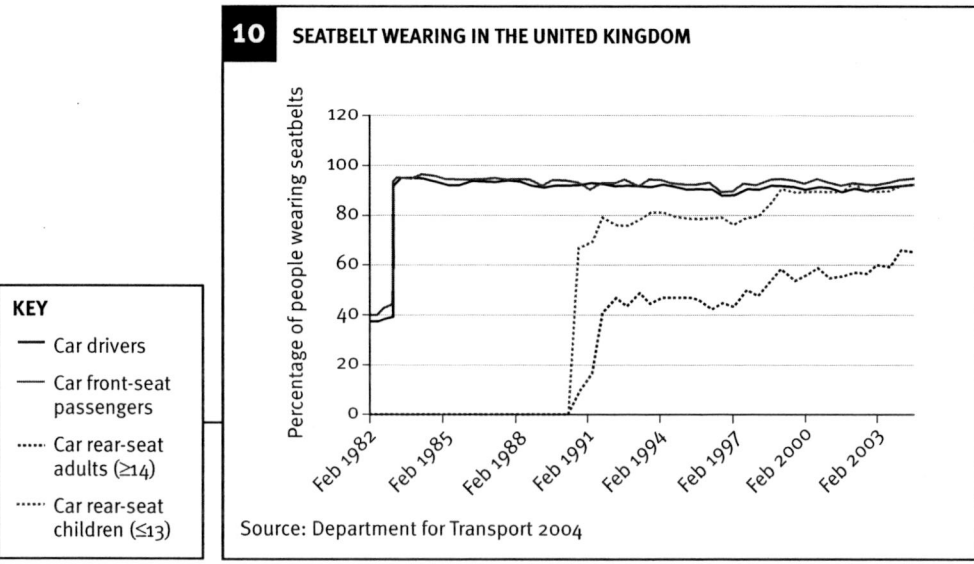

10 SEATBELT WEARING IN THE UNITED KINGDOM

KEY
— Car drivers
— Car front-seat passengers
····· Car rear-seat adults (≥14)
······ Car rear-seat children (≤13)

Source: Department for Transport 2004

This has had an impact on fatalities and injuries. Studies comparing accident data in the year before and the year after the first seatbelt legislation found fatalities were down by between 23 and 32 per cent; the number of patients brought to hospital declined by 15 per cent; and those requiring admission to wards dropped by 25 per cent (Hobbs 1978; Rutherford, Greenfield *et al* 1985). Several studies found that there were fewer patients with severe injuries, although there were more with bruising and neck sprains. Seatbelt wearers did suffer major brain injuries, but the severity of injuries in unbelted drivers and passengers was worse (Tunbridge 1989; Harvey and Durbin 1986; Bradbury and Robertson 1993).

Some researchers have suggested that the impact of seatbelts on fatalities was less than advocates of mandatory seatbelts had hoped for, and that when drivers felt safer, they took more risks (Adams 1985a, 1985b; McCarthy 1989). Other researchers noted that injured patients not wearing a seatbelt were more likely to be male, young and intoxicated – the group least responsive to government policies. It was uneven adoption of seatbelts, they argued, that explained the modest impact on fatalities (Dee 1998).

Despite these controversies, road safety organisations believe that since 1983, mandatory seatbelt use has prevented 50,000 deaths, 590,000 serious casualties and 1,590,000 minor injuries (Department for Transport 2001). The savings made as a result of these avoided deaths and injuries – in terms of medical and emergency care, lost economic output, and loss of life and injury – is estimated at £163 billion (Department for Transport 2003b).

BAC LIMITS
UK and international studies show that introducing blood-alcohol limits has an impact on fatalities and casualties. A US study based on data from 50 states found that fatalities declined by 14 per cent between 1980 and 1997 when the legal blood-alcohol concentration level dropped from 0.10 per cent to 0.08 per cent (Grube 2004).

Conversely, when the blood-alcohol concentration limit was increased from 0.02 per cent to 0.05 per cent in Portugal, fatalities increased by 10 per cent (Eurocare 2003).

A survey of US and Australian studies showed that introducing stricter limits for novice drivers reduced fatal crashes by between 9 per cent and 24 per cent, and injuries by between 4 per cent and 17 per cent (Waller, Naidoo *et al* 2002).

Figure 11 shows the link between blood-alcohol concentration limits and fatalities in alcohol-related accidents. The United Kingdom's blood-alcohol limit is higher than the 0.05 per cent that is common in mainland Europe, but its casualty rate is lower than other countries with the same blood-alcohol limit.

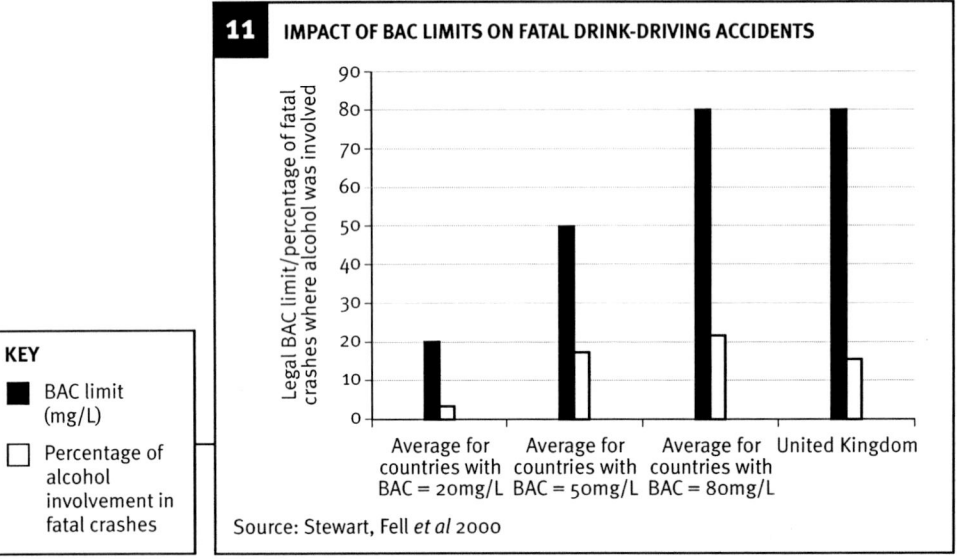

11   **IMPACT OF BAC LIMITS ON FATAL DRINK-DRIVING ACCIDENTS**

KEY

■ BAC limit (mg/L)

□ Percentage of alcohol involvement in fatal crashes

Source: Stewart, Fell *et al* 2000

SURVEILLANCE

The high compliance rates for seatbelts and drink-driving are a result of drivers' and passengers' perceptions of the risk of getting caught and fear of the likely legal penalties.

From 1992 to 1994, there were, on average, 120,000 fixed penalty notices, written cautions and court prosecutions for not wearing a seatbelt. By 2000, this had risen to over 200,000, even though the number of seatbelt wearers had risen in this period. This suggests that surveillance had increased (Department for Transport 2003a).

Since 1996, drivers involved in accidents have been breathalysed. Even though the number of roadside screening tests increased from 450,000 in 1988 to 815,000 in 1998, the percentage of positive (and refused tests) has fallen from nearly 25 per cent to 12 per cent, indicating that fewer people are drinking and driving (Clayton and Tunbridge 2000). The percentage of drivers involved in car accidents who have tested positive has also fallen (*see* Figure 12, opposite).

A survey showed that respondents restricted their drinking for fear of being breathalysed, even though they realised their chances of being stopped were small, and their knowledge of the penalties was poor (Lennox and Quimby 1990).

Random or selective testing, although not permitted in the United Kingdom, has proven effective in Australia, New Zealand, the United States and some European countries in reducing fatalities. On average, random testing resulted in an 18 per cent decrease in alcohol-related crashes and a 22 per cent decrease in fatal crashes, while selective breath testing resulted in a 20 per cent reduction in crashes and a 23 per cent reduction in fatal crashes (Waller, Naidoo *et al* 2002).

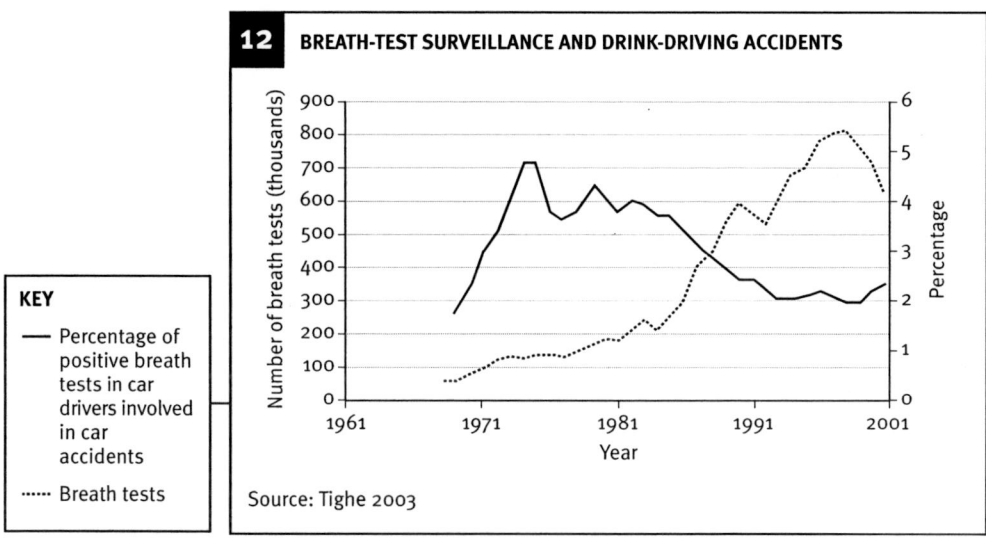

12 BREATH-TEST SURVEILLANCE AND DRINK-DRIVING ACCIDENTS

Source: Tighe 2003

EDUCATION

Attitudes to wearing seatbelts and drink-driving have shifted over the past 30 years and long-running education campaigns have played a part. Public opinion surveys show that people believe that seatbelts are protective; 98 per cent of those questioned in a 2003 survey rated not wearing a front seatbelt as 'very' or 'fairly dangerous' (Department for Transport 2003a; Quimby and Downing 1991).

Isolated road-safety campaigns are relatively ineffective in changing behaviour. From 1975 to 1982, the government ran annual education campaigns to encourage drivers and passengers to wear seatbelts, with little success – about 30 per cent of drivers used seatbelts (Mackay 1987; McCarthy 1989). Compliance soared when seatbelts became mandatory.

Education campaigns also need to be continual. In the early 1970s, drink-driving education campaigns ceased for a few years, and the proportion of road fatalities involving alcohol rose from 15 per cent in 1967 to 35 per cent in 1975. Since 1977, drink-driving education campaigns have been run every year, and by 1999 just 4 per cent of people involved in road accidents failed the breath test (Royal Society for the Prevention of Accidents 2005).

Indeed, drinking and driving is no longer acceptable, even if one drives 'safely'. In 1979, 51 per cent of people polled had driven after drinking at least once in the previous week. By 1997, this had dropped to 23 per cent. The percentage drinking six or more units and then driving fell from 15 per cent to 3 per cent (Lennox and Quimby 1990; Royal Society for the Prevention of Accidents 2005; Scottish Executive Social Research 2004).

Summary

The story of road safety, like smoking, is one of increasing regulation. Research shows that government legislation for mandatory seatbelts and alcohol limits for drivers have resulted in individual behavioural change and reduced fatalities and casualties from road accidents. Public education campaigns were relatively ineffective until backed by legal penalties to enforce compliance, and together, both interventions have changed attitudes to seatbelt wearing and safety.

Conclusions

The case studies on alcohol, smoking and road safety show that state intervention goes through phases of regulation and liberalisation. What is striking is that from a long-term historical perspective, governments intervene in a laggardly way. Governments come under pressure from powerful industrial interests to maintain the status quo. Britain, like other governments internationally, was, for a long time, reluctant to take on the tobacco industry, and today it also faces a strong alcohol and food lobby. It also takes time for scientific knowledge about particular risks to be accepted as part of mainstream thought and begin to influence policy. So it took 27 years before seatbelts became mandatory, while medical evidence about smoking has been clear for the past 60 years, but the government has been timid about regulation. The link between air pollution and respiratory disease was also well known long before the government introduced legislation. There are innumerable examples showing that governments are reluctant to act in a precautionary way on emerging scientific evidence about health, because they fear action will be too expensive and offend industrial interests (Harremoes, Gee *et al* 2001).

What brings about change is political pressure and cultural change. Pressure groups influence government and shape public opinion. The temperance movement campaigned against drinking (*see* p 11) while modern lobby groups, such as ASH have campaigned for stronger controls on smoking (*see* p 19). Without these campaigns, it is arguable whether governments of the time would have acted in the way they did. These interest groups helped create and reflected changes in cultural attitudes.

Almost every government intervention in the public health arena has been criticised by critics of the time as a sign of tyranny, nanny statism, or the end of individual freedom. We suggested at the beginning of the paper that 'stewardship' might be a more appropriate way to understand the fiscal and regulatory codes governments use to shape behaviour. True, such intervention might limit individual freedom a little, but in return intervention brings benefits to individuals and society. As a result, some political theorists argue that government intervention is not inconsistent with individual freedom. Sunstein and Thaler (2003), for example, suggest that public policy eliminates obviously bad choices and encourages more positive ones to promote individual and general well-being. Goodin (1995) believes that where people have a conscious desire to do something they cannot bring themselves to do, public policy can enable them to recognise and act on their desire.

Certainly, the historical and contemporary evidence discussed in Part 2 illustrates the considerable individual and public health benefits of once-contested interventions – results which arguably mitigate the small limitations on individual freedom and choice. The findings from Part 2 show the positive impact of education, taxation and restrictive legislation on shaping individuals' choices for healthier behaviour, and ultimately on health.

Education

The case studies show that education campaigns are consistently popular. They are cheap and cost effective, and raise awareness about the health impact of particular problems. However, evidence suggests that awareness does not translate into changed behaviour. Adolescents do not smoke or drink less following health education programmes (*see* pp 14–15, 22), and until it became mandatory, drivers were unwilling to follow the advice of safety education campaigns and use their seatbelts (*see* p 27).

Education and awareness raising have a role in explaining health risks, justifying interventions, and creating new social norms, but they need to be backed by regulatory and fiscal measures if the aim is to change behaviour.

Taxation

Innumerable studies show that taxation shapes consumption patterns and this affects health. Increase the price of tobacco, keep taxes in line with inflation and living standards, and smokers smoke less, or even quit (*see* p 20). Let alcohol prices drop in relation to incomes, let taxes lag, and consumption rises (*see* p 13). Taxation is universally effective, although it does have a disproportionate effect on poorer income groups.

Restrictive measures

The case studies suggest that restrictive measures are particularly effective at improving public health, since regulations shape the framework within which individual choices are made, and potential penalties ensure compliance. Legislation can also affect issues that individuals on their own can do little to control, and sets frameworks that promote changes in the whole population.

Cross-country surveys show that total advertising bans on tobacco and alcohol reduce consumption and associated mortality levels (*see* pp 14, 21). Laws that reduce the availability of alcohol and tobacco reduce consumption and associated health problems (*see* p 14, 21).

The law mandating seatbelts saw a dramatic rise in seatbelt use that long-running education campaigns had been unable to achieve (*see* p 24). Similarly, the threat of being breathalysed is sufficient to persuade most people to control their drinking if they are planning to drive.

Impact on inequalities

However the benefits of government intervention are not spread evenly across high- and low-income socio-economic groups.

Alcohol-related mortality was higher in higher-income groups and smoking was evenly spread across all social groups in the immediate post-war period. But today, poorer social groups are more likely to die early and suffer from chronic conditions as a result of smoking and drinking. This suggests that rich and poor have not responded to fiscal and regulatory measures in the same way.

The shift in alcohol-related mortality, for example, may indicate that higher incomes and lower alcohol taxes have made alcohol more available to poorer social groups than it was previously. Or it may reflect lower levels of awareness about the problems caused by drinking, since surveys show that lower-income social classes are usually less aware of health education messages.

It may also reflect the impact of increasing economic and social inequality on health (Sassi 2005; Shaw, Davey Smith *et al* 2005). Some researchers suggest that economic insecurity, social isolation, and lack of optimism about personal health and future prospects make it more difficult for individuals from disadvantaged backgrounds to make positive health choices and change lifestyles.

These shortcomings have encouraged interest in targeted interventions to reduce inequalities, yet evidence suggests that these are less effective than universal ones, and stigmatise recipients and undermine social trust and cohesion (Rothstein and Uslaner 2005). Certainly, legislation that improves the quality of resources used by everyone, such as environmental and air quality standards, tend to have a greater positive impact on poorer, more deprived areas, which are usually more polluted.

Despite the difficulty of reducing health inequalities through education, taxation and regulation – which suggests the cause is deeply rooted in socio-economic inequalities – the individual and social benefits of government intervention are clear. Should we then argue that the ends justify the means? Probably not, as this could open the door to highly coercive measures. Imagine police cautions to smoking and drinking pregnant women, or to mothers of bottle-fed babies or even raids to ensure safe sex is being practised (apartheid South Africa banned sexual relationships across the colour line, and gay and lesbian relationships were illegal in many countries until recently, so this is not beyond the bounds of possibility!).

But it is worth considering the philosophical discussion that underlies the rhetoric of the nanny-state debate about the role of government, the limits to government intervention, and the conditions under which intervention is acceptable.

At the outset of this paper, we suggested that 'stewardship' might be a more appropriate term than 'nanny statism' to understand the justification for and impact of the range of interventions that governments use to shape behaviour. Public health measures that set new social standards and bring about changes that individuals on their own cannot make, fall easily into the stewardship framework. They are measures that promote the public good.

Stewardship also implies that a government protects its citizens against harm from others. We accept that laws against murder allow us to live in relative safety, and laws against fraud allow us to enter economic contracts. And few would quibble with government regulations protecting vulnerable individuals, such as children, or a society against polluting or corrupt industries. Similarly, laws against drink-driving, speed limits or smoking in public places help protect us from the potentially dangerous actions of others by defining what is acceptable and ensuring compliance through penalties, surveillance and social pressure.

Stewardship is more controversial when it comes to protecting individuals from harming themselves rather than others. However, we try to protect individuals wanting to commit suicide, from acting on their desire, knowing that they might feel differently about their lives in future. Are smoking, drinking and eating unhealthily any different? Governments cannot ban these activities, nor can it compel people to do things they do not wish to. But the case studies suggest they can encourage better choices through regulation, taxation, advertising codes and informational campaigns. These may restrict individual choices a little, but they also make it easier for individuals to make healthier choices if they wish. Many smokers want to quit. Many overweight people would like to be thinner. And few would welcome a bout of syphilis or chlamydia from a night of unprotected sex. If government interventions make it easier for individuals to act on these desires, then it is difficult to argue that it undermines their liberty. Rather government stewardship sets the framework for encouraging healthier decisions.

The proposals for the partial smoking ban and for food labelling are now being discussed at national and EU levels. There are many people and organisations opposing these plans, and many who feel that they do not go far enough. What is evident from our historical surveys is that this debate is part of the process of changing attitudes. A decade from now some of these laws will be in place and go unnoticed in our daily lives, others will still be contested. The process reflects the way some scientific knowledge about risks to health becomes an acceptable part of mainstream thought and action. It is also part of a political debate over where to draw the line on government intervention and individual responsibility and the role of government as a steward for public health.

References

Action on Smoking and Health (2004a). *Factsheet No 2: Smoking statistics: illness and death.* ASH website. Available at: www.ash.org.uk (accessed on 5 September 2005)

Action on Smoking and Health (2004b). *Factsheet No 14: Smoking in workplaces and public places.* ASH website. Available at: www.ash.org.uk (accessed on 5 September 2005)

Action on Smoking and Health (2004c). *Factsheet No 19: Tobacco advertising and promotion.* ASH website. Available at: www.ash.org.uk (accessed on 5 September 2005)

Action on Smoking and Health (2004d). *ASH Briefing: The UK ban on tobacco advertising.* ASH website. Available at: www.ash.org.uk (accessed on 5 September 2005)

Action on Smoking and Health (2002). *Basic Facts Three: Tobacco economics.* ASH website. Available at: www.ash.org.uk (accessed on 5 September 2005)

Action on Smoking and Health, Health Development Agency (2003). *Smoking and Health Inequalities.* National Institute for Health and Clinical Excellence website. Available at: www.publichealth.nice.org.uk/download.aspx?o=502021 (accessed on 5 September 2005)

Action on Smoking and Health, Health Development Agency (2001). *Smoking and Health Inequalities.* National Institute for Health and Clinical Excellence website. Available at: www.publichealth.nice.org.uk/page.aspx?o=502021 (accessed on 5 September 2005)

Adams J (1985a). 'Smeed's Law, seat belts, and the emperor's new clothes' in *Human Behaviour and Traffic Safety*, Evans L and Schwing RW eds, pp 193–248. New York and London: Plenum Press.

Adams J (1985b). *Risk and Freedom: The record of road safety regulation.* Cardiff: Transport Publishing Projects.

Ashby E, Anderson M (1981). *The Politics of Clean Air.* Oxford: Clarendon Press.

Babor T, Caetano R, Casswell S, Edwards G, Giesbrecht N, Graham K, Grube JW, Grunewald P, Hill L, Holder HD (2003). *Alcohol – No Ordinary Commodity: Research and public policy.* Oxford: Oxford University Press.

Baker A, Rooney C (2003). 'Recent trends in alcohol-related mortality, and the impact of ICD-10 on the monitoring of these deaths in England and Wales'. *Office for National Statistics Health Statistics Quarterly*, vol 17, pp 5–14.

Berridge V (1998). 'Science and policy: the case of post-war British smoking policy' in *Ashes to Ashes: The history of smoking and health*, Lock S, Reynolds L and Tansey EM eds, pp 143–63. Atlanta: Rodopi.

Biener L, Harris JE, Hamilton W (2000). 'Impact of the Massachusetts tobacco control programme: population based trend analysis'. *British Medical Journal*, vol 321, no 7257, pp 351–54.

Bradbury A, Robertson C (1993). 'Prospective audit of the pattern, severity and circumstances of injury sustained by vehicle occupants as a result of road traffic accidents'. *Archives of Emergency Medicine*, vol 10, no 1, pp 15–23.

Brimblecombe P (1987). *The Big Smoke: A history of air pollution in London since medieval times.* London: Methuen.

Bristow J (2004). 'A really bad habit'. Spiked-online, 12 March. Available at: www.spiked-online.com/ Printable?0000000CA473.htm (accessed on 5 September 2005)

Burnett J (1999). *Liquid Pleasures: A social history of drinks in modern Britain.* London, New York: Routledge.

Cabinet Office (2004). *Alcohol Harm Reduction Strategy for England.* London: The Stationery Office.

Cabinet Office Strategy Unit (2003). *Interim Analytical Report for the National Alcohol Harm Reduction Strategy 2003.* London: The Stationery Office.

Canadian Cancer Society (2001). *Compilation of Selected Evidence Regarding the Impact of Higher Tobacco Prices on Tobacco Use: A submission prepared for the House of Commons Standing Committee on Finance.* Toronto: Canadian Cancer Society. Available at: www.globalink.org/tobacco/ docs/economics/200109ccs-priceimpact.htm (accessed on 5 September 2005)

Casswell S, Pledger M, Pratap S (2002). 'Trajectories of drinking from 18 to 26 years: identification and prediction'. *Addiction*, vol 97, pp 1427–37.

Casswell S, Zhang J-F (1998). 'Impact of liking for advertising and brand allegiance on drinking and alcohol-related aggression: a longitudinal study'. *Addiction*, vol 93, no 8, pp 1209–17.

Centre for History in Public Health, London School of Hygiene and Tropical Medicine (2002). *The Big Smoke: Fifty years after the 1952 London Smog – a commemorative conference.* LSHTM website. Available at: www.lshtm.ac.uk/history/bigsmoke.html (accessed on 5 September 2005)

Chaloupka F, Grossman H, Saffer H (2002). *The Effects of Price on Alcohol Consumption and Alcohol-related Problems.* National Institute on Alcohol Abuse and Alcoholism website. Available at: www. niaaa.nih.gov/publications/arh26-1/22-34.htm (accessed on 5 September 2005)

Clayton AB, Tunbridge RJ (2000). *Drinking and Driving in Great Britain: The end of the decline?* Paper prepared for presentation at T2000, the 15th International Conference on Alcohol, Drugs and Traffic Safety, Stockholm, Sweden.

Crosbie D, Stockwell T, Wodak A, Ferrall I (2000). *Alcohol, Taxation Reform and Public Health in Australia: A submission to the Federal Parliamentary Enquiry into substance abuse in Australian Communities.* Parliament of Australia, House of Representatives website. Available at: www.aph.gov. au/house/committee/fca/subabuse/sub123.pdf (accessed on 5 September 2005)

Daily Mail (2001). 'Labour launches manifesto'. *Daily Mail*, 16 May. Available at: www.dailymail.co. uk/pages/live/articles/news/news.html?in_article_id=46508&in_page_id=1770 (accessed on 5 September 2005)

Dee T (1998). 'Reconsidering the effects of seat belt laws and their enforcement status'. *Accident Analysis and Prevention*, vol 30, no 1, pp 1–10.

Department of Health (2004). *Choosing Health: Making healthy choices easier.* London: The Stationery Office.

Department of Health (2003). *Statistics on Smoking: England.* Statistical Bulletin 2003/21. London: Department of Health.

Department of Health (1998a). *Smoking Kills: A white paper on tobacco*. London: The Stationery Office.

Department of Health (1998b). *Statistics on Smoking: England 1976–1996*. Statistical Bulletin 1998/25. London: Department of Health.

Department of Health and Office for National Statistics (2004). *Statistics on Alcohol: England*. Statistical Bulletin 2004/15. London: Department of Health.

Department for Transport (2004). 'Road safety statistics: Great Britain car and van seat belt wearing – percentage rates (October 2004)'. Think! Road Safety website. Available at: www.thinkroadsafety. gov.uk/statistics/belt0410.htm (accessed 5 September 2005)

Department for Transport (2003a). *Attitudes to Road Safety*. Department for Transport website. Available at: www.dft.gov.uk/stellent/groups/dft_transstats/documents/page/dft_transstats _028383.hcsp (accessed on 5 September 2005)

Department for Transport (2003b). *Highways Economics Note No 1: 2002*. Department for Transport website. Available at: www.dft.gov.uk/stellent/groups/dft_rdsafety/documents/page/dft_ rdsafety_026183.hcsp (accessed on 5 September 2005)

Department for Transport (2003c). *Road Casualties in Great Britain 2003: Annual Report*. Department for Transport website. Available at: www.dft.gov.uk/stellent/groups/dft_control/documents/ contentservertemplate/dft_index.hcst?n=11541&l=3 (accessed on 5 September 2005)

Department for Transport (2001). 'Seatbelt Facts – Laws passed and lives saved: 20 facts for the 20th anniversary of compulsory seatbelt wearing'. Think! Seatbelts website. Available at: www. thinkseatbelts.com (accessed 5 September 2005)

Department for Transport (2000). *Tomorrow's Roads: Safer for everyone*. London: Department for Transport. Available at: www.dft.gov.uk/stellent/groups/dft_rdsafety/documents/page/dft_ rdsafety_504644-02.hcsp#P86_3774 (accessed on 5 September 2005)

Drever F, Whitehead M eds (1997). *Health Inequalities: Decennial supplement*. Series DS, no 15, pp 1–257. London: The Stationery Office.

Dyer O (2004). 'One million people die on the world's roads every year'. *British Medical Journal*, vol 328, p 851.

Edwards G, Anderson P, Babor TF, Casswell S, Ferrence R, Giesbrecht N, Godfrey C, Holder HD, Lemmens PHMM, Mäkelä K, Midanik LT, Narström T, Österberg E, Romelsjö A, Room R, Simpura J, Skog OJ (1994). 'Retail price influences on alcohol consumption and taxation of alcohol as a prevention strategy' in *Alcohol Policy and the Public Good*. Oxford: Oxford University Press.

Eisner MD, Smith AK, Blanc PO (1998). 'Bartenders' respiratory health after establishment of smoke-free bars and taverns'. *Journal of the American Medical Association*, vol 280, no 22, pp 1909–14.

Eurocare (2003). *Drinking and Driving in Europe: A Eurocare report to the European Union*. Brussels: Eurocare.

Fairclough N (2000). *New Labour, New Language?* London: Routledge.

Farrelly MC, Nonnemaker JM, Chou R, Hyland A, Peterson KK, Bauer UE (2005). 'Changes in hospitality workers' exposure to secondhand smoke following the implementation of New York's smoke-free law'. *Tobacco Control*, vol 14, pp 236–41.

Fichtenberg CM, Glantz SA (2002). 'Effect of smoke-free workplaces on smoking behaviour: systematic review'. *British Medical Journal*, vol 325, no 7357, pp 188–94.

Future Foundation (2005). *The Assault on Pleasure*. Future Foundation website. Available at: www.futurefoundation.net/Assault_on_pleasure.html (accessed on 5 September 2005)

Glover S (2004). 'Why, for once, the nanny state is right'. *Daily Mail*, 6 July.

Godfrey C (1997). 'Can tax be used to minimise harm? A health economist's perspective' in *Alcohol: Minimising the harm – what works?*, Plant M, Single E and Stockwell T eds, pp 29–42. London: Free Association Books.

Goodin R (1995). 'In defense of the nanny state' in *Rights and the Common Good: The communitarian perspective*, Etzioni A ed, pp 123–38. New York: St Martins Press.

Grey A, Owen L, Bolling K (2000). *A Breath of Fresh Air: Tackling smoking through the media*. London: Health Development Agency.

Grube J (2004). 'Preventing alcohol-related problems: alcohol policy challenges' in *Putting Research Into Action: A Symposium on the Implementation of Research-Based Impaired Driving Counter Measures*. Washington DC: Transportation Research Board. Available at: www.trb.org (accessed on 5 September 2005)

Harremoes P, Gee D, MacGarvin M, Stirling A, Keys J, Wynne B, Vaz SG (2001). *Late Lessons from Early Warnings: The precautionary principle 1896–2000*. Environmental Report 22. Copenhagen: European Environment Agency.

Harrison B (1971). *Drink and the Victorians: The temperance question in England 1815–1872*. London: Faber and Faber.

Harrison L, Gardiner E (1999). 'Do the rich really die young? Alcohol-related mortality and social class in Great Britain, 1988–94'. *Addiction*, vol 94, no 12, pp 1871–80.

Harvey AC, Durbin J (1986). 'The effects of seat belt legislation on British road casualties: a case study in structural time series modelling'. *Journal of the Royal Statistical Society Series A*, vol 149, pp 187–227.

Health Development Agency (2004). *Smoking Interventions with Children and Young People*. HDA Briefing No 6. National Institute for Health and Clinical Excellence website. Available at: www.publichealth.nice.org.uk/download.aspx?o=502773 (accessed on 5 September 2005)

Hilton M (2000). *Smoking in British Popular Culture 1800–2000*. Manchester: Manchester University Press.

Hobbs CA (1978). *The Effectiveness of Seat Belts in Reducing Injuries to Car Occupants*. Transport and Road Research Laboratory report 811. Crowthorne: TRRL.

House of Commons (1981–82). 'House of Commons official report: sixth series'. *Parliamentary Debates: Commons*, vol 28, pp 633–40.

International Study of Alcohol Control Experiences, World Health Organisation Regional Office for Europe (1981). *Alcohol, Society and the State: A comparative study of alcohol control, vol 1*. Toronto: Addiction Research Foundation.

Jarvis MJ, Wardle J, Waller J, Owen L (2003). 'Prevalence of hardcore smokers in England and associated attitudes and beliefs: cross sectional study'. *British Medical Journal*, vol 326, p 1061.

Jha P, Chaloupka F (2000). 'The Economics of Global Tobacco Control'. *British Medical Journal*, vol 321, pp 358–61.

Kennedy C (2003). 'Bye, bye to big government'. Speech to the Social Market Foundation, 15 July. Available at: www.libdems.org.uk/index.cfm/page.homepage/section.home/article.4976 (accessed on 5 September 2005)

Lancaster T, Stead L, Silagy C, Sowden A (2000). 'Effectiveness of interventions to help people stop smoking: findings from the Cochrane Library'. *British Medical Journal*, vol 321, pp 355–8.

Leichter H (1986). 'Lives, liberty and seat belts in Britain: lessons for the United States'. *International Journal of Health Services*, vol 16, no 2, pp 213–26.

Lennox R, Quimby A (1990). *Survey of Drink-driving Behaviour, Knowledge and Attitudes*. Crowthorne: Transport and Road Research Laboratory.

Liberal Democrats (2004). 'Obesity report: urgency and determination needed from government'. Liberal Democrats website. Available at: www.libdems.org.uk/index.cfm/page.homepage/section. home/article.6855 (accessed on 5 September 2005)

Luckhurst T (2004). 'Warning: The nanny state can seriously damage your enjoyment of life'. *Daily Mail*, 25 June.

Mackay M (1987). 'Seat belt legislation in Britain'. *Journal of Trauma*, vol 27, no 7, pp 759–62.

Marmot M, Feeney A (1999). 'Inequality, alcohol and alcohol-associated harm' in *Inequalities in Health: A series of seminars held by the Health Education Authority*, Waller S, Crosier A and McVey D eds, pp 79–85. London: Health Education Authority.

McCarthy M (1989). 'The benefit of seat belt legislation in the United Kingdom'. *Journal of Epidemiology and Community Health*, vol 43, pp 218–22.

Melihan-Cheinin P, Hirsch A (1997). 'Effects of smoke-free environments, advertising bans and price increases' in *The Tobacco Epidemic*, Boliger CT and Fagestroem KP eds, pp 230–46. Basel: Kargar.

Miller N (2005). 'Statement of Nancy Miller, Ph.D., CHES Assistant Commissioner Bureau of Tobacco Control before the New York City Council Committee on Health regarding Evaluation of the Tobacco Use, Prevention and Control Program'. Testimony, 9 February. The New York City Department of Health and Mental Hygiene website. Available at: www.nyc.gov/html/doh/html/testi/ testi20050209.shtml (accessed on 5 September 2005)

Mosedale J, Francis L, Clarkson E (2003). 'Drinking and driving' in *Road Casualties in Great Britain 2003: Annual Report*. Department for Transport website. Available at: www.dft.gov.uk/stellent/ groups/dft_control/documents/contentservertemplate/dft_index.hcst?n=11541&l=3 (accessed on 5 September 2005)

Naidoo B, Warm D, Quigley R, Taylor R (2004). *Smoking and Public Health: A review of interventions to increase smoking cessation, reduce smoking initiation and prevent further uptake of smoking*. London: Health Development Agency.

Office for National Statistics (2003). *Smoking Related Behaviour and Attitudes, 2003*. London: The Stationery Office.

Olsson O, Wikstrom P (1982). 'Effects of the experimental Saturday closing of liquor retail stores in Sweden'. *Contemporary Drug Problems*, vol 1, no 3, pp 325–54.

Opinion Leader Research (2004). *Public Attitudes to Public Health Policy*. London: King's Fund.

Peto R (1994). 'Smoking and death: the past 40 years and the next 40'. *British Medical Journal (International edition)*, vol 309, no 6959, p 937.

Peto R, Darby S, Deo H, Silcocks P, Whitley E, Doll R (2000). 'Smoking, smoking cessation and lung cancer in the UK since 1950: combination of national statistics with two case-control studies'. *British Medical Journal*, vol 321, pp 323–29.

Plant MA (1997). 'Trends in alcohol and illicit drug-related diseases' in *The Health of Adult Britain 1841–1994, vol 1*, Charlton J and Murphy M, pp 114–27. London: The Stationery Office.

Pollard S (2003). 'Smoking bans are offensive. But they work'. *The Independent*, 27 October.

Pollock D (1992). *Denial and Delay: The political history of smoking and health, 1951–1964*. London: Action on Smoking and Health.

Porter D (1999). *Health, Civilisation and the State: A history of public health from ancient to modern times*. London: Routledge.

The Portman Group (2001). *Alcohol and Society: Research study conducted by MORI for The Portman Group*. London: The Portman Group.

Quimby A, Downing C (1991). *Road Users' Attitudes to Some Road Safety and Transportation Issues*. Transport and Road Research Laboratory report 227. Crowthorne: TRRL.

Raistrick D, Hodgson R, Ritson B (1999). *Tackling Alcohol Together: The evidence base for a UK alcohol policy*. London: Free Association Books.

Richardson K (2001). *Smoking, Low Income and Health Inequalities: Thematic discussion document*. Action on Smoking and Health website. Available at: www.ash.org.uk/html/policy/discussion.html (accessed on 5 September 2005)

Rose L (1984). *Drink and Drugs*. London: Batsford Academic and Educational.

Rothstein B, Uslaner E (2005). *All for All: Equality and social trust*. London School of Economics health and social care discussion paper no 15. London: LSE.

Royal Society for the Prevention of Accidents (2005). *Drinking and Driving Policy Paper*. ROSPA website. Available at: www.rospa.com/roadsafety/info/drink_drive.pdf (accessed on 5 September 2005)

Rutherford WH, Greenfield T, Hayes HRM, Nelson JK (1985). *The Medical Effects of Seat Belt Legislation in the United Kingdom*. Department of Health and Social Security research report no 13. London: HMSO.

Saffer H (1991). 'Alcohol advertising bans and alcohol abuse: an international perspective'. *Journal of Health Economics*, vol 10, pp 65–79.

Saffer H, Chaloupka F (2000). 'The effect of tobacco advertising bans on tobacco consumption'. *Journal of Health Economics*, vol 19, pp 1117–37.

Saltman RB, Ferroussier-Davis O (2000). 'The concept of stewardship in health policy'. *Bulletin of the World Health Organisation*, vol 78, no 6, pp 732–39.

Sassi F (2005). 'Tackling health inequalities' in *A More Equal Society? New Labour, poverty, inequality and exclusion*, Hills J and Stewart K, pp 69–92. Bristol: Policy Press.

Scottish Executive (2004). *Opinion Survey: Smoking*. Scottish Executive website. Available at: www.scotland.gov.uk/Topics/Health/health/smoking/Opinion-Survey (accessed on 5 September 2005)

Scottish Executive Social Research (2004). *Scottish Executive Evaluation of the 2003–2004 Festive Drink Drive Campaign*. Scottish Executive website. Available at: www.scotland.gov.uk/library5/transport/fddc-00.asp (accessed on 5 September 2005)

Scottish Executive Social Research (2003). *Omnibus Survey: Testing public opinion on licensing law and alcohol consumption*. Edinburgh: SESR.

Shaw M, Davey Smith G, Dorling D (2005). 'Health inequalities and New Labour: how the promises compare with real progress'. *British Medical Journal*, vol 330, pp 1016–21.

Starr S (2004). 'Exercise in futility'. Spiked-online website. Available at: www.spiked-online.com/Printable/0000000CA508.htm (accessed on 5 September 2005)

Stewart K, Fell J, Ellison-Potter P, Seedler B (2000). *International Comparisons of Laws and Alcohol Crash Rates: Lessons learned*. Paper presented at International Conference on Alcohol, Drugs and Traffic Safety, Stockholm, Sweden. International Council on Alcohol, Drugs and Traffic Safety website. Available at: www.icadts.org/proceedings/show.php?paper=2000-132 (accessed on 5 September 2005)

Sunstein CS, Thaler RH (2003). *Libertarian Paternalism is Not an Oxymoron*. AEI-Brookings working paper 03–2. Chicago: University of Chicago.

Taylor K, Fraser S (2002). 'Eat unhealthily in the name of democracy'. *Scotland on Sunday*, 25 August.

Taylor P (1984). *Smoke Ring: The politics of tobacco*. London: Bodley Head.

The Guardian, editorial (2004). 'Fit for purpose'. *The Guardian*, 1 May.

Tighe A ed (2003). *Statistical Handbook*. London: Brewing Publications Limited.

Tobacco Information and Prevention Source (2004). *World Health Organisation: Europe – United Kingdom of Great Britain and Northern Ireland*. Centre for Chronic Disease Prevention and Health Promotion website. Available at: www.cdc.gov/tobacco/who/unitedki.htm (accessed on 5 September 2005)

Townsend J, Roderick P, Cooper J (1994). 'Cigarette smoking by socioeconomic group, sex and age: effects of price, income and health publicity'. *British Medical Journal*, vol 309, pp 923–27.

Tunbridge RJ (1989). *The Long Term Effect of Seat Belt Legislation on Road User Injury Patterns*. Transport and Road Research Laboratory research report 239. Crowthorne: TRRL.

Waller S, Naidoo B, Thom B (2002). *Prevention and Reduction of Alcohol Misuse: Evidence briefing.* London: Health Development Agency.

Wanless D (2004). *Securing Good Health for the Whole Population: Final report.* London: HMSO.

World Bank (2001). *Economics of Tobacco Control: Myths and facts.* World Bank website. Available at: www.worldbank.org/tobacco/faq.asp (accessed on 5 September 2005)

Whitehead M (1987). *The Health Divide: Inequalities in Health in the 1980s.* London: Health Education Authority.

In the past year, there has been much debate over the government's
role in public health issues such as smoking and obesity. Is government
intervention in these areas an example of 'nanny statism' – an
unnecessary intrusion into people's lives? Or is it a form of 'stewardship'
– part of government's responsibility to protect national health? This
paper looks at the options open to governments that want to influence
individual and collective behaviour to reduce health risks. It also
examines historical and contemporary evidence on the impact of
state intervention on public health.

ISBN 1-85717-538-7

9 781857 175387

£6·50